# ADVANCEMENTS IN BREAST CANCER RESEARCH

*A Comprehensive Overview*

Dr. Bernd Kortig

**ADVANCEMENTS IN BREAST CANCER RESEARCH**

# TABLE OF CONTENTS

*Introduction to Breast Cancer: Epidemiology, Incidence, and Mortality Trends*

*Etiology and Risk Factors: Genetic, Environmental, and Lifestyle Influences*

*Biology of Breast Cancer: Oncogenes, Tumor Suppressor Genes, and Signaling Pathways*

**ADVANCEMENTS IN BREAST CANCER RESEARCH**

*Breast Anatomy and Physiology: Normal Development and Function*

*Pathology of Breast Cancer: Histological Subtypes and Molecular Classification*

*Early Detection and Screening Strategies: Mammography, MRI, Ultrasound, and Biomarkers*

*Tumor Microenvironment: Role of Stromal Cells, Immune Cells, and Extracellular Matrix*

**ADVANCEMENTS IN BREAST CANCER RESEARCH**

## Metastasis: Mechanisms, Key Players, and Therapeutic Targets

## Animal Models

## Imaging Techniques in Breast Cancer Diagnosis and Monitoring

## Biomarkers in Breast Cancer: Prognostic, Predictive, and Therapeutic Targets

## Testing and Counseling: BRCA Mutations and Beyond

**ADVANCEMENTS IN BREAST CANCER RESEARCH**

*Therapies in Breast Cancer: HER2-Targeted Agents, Hormonal Therapies, and PARP Inhibitors*

*Mechanisms of Action, Resistance, and Novel Approaches in Breast Cancer Treatment*

*Radiation Therapy: Techniques, Fractionation Schedules, and Side Effects*

*Immunotherapy in Breast Cancer: Checkpoint Inhibitors, CAR-T Cells, and Vaccines*

**ADVANCEMENTS IN BREAST CANCER RESEARCH**

*Precision Medicine in Breast Cancer Treatment: Molecular Profiling and Personalized Therapies*

*Clinical Trials in Breast Cancer: Design, Implementation, and Ethical Considerations*

*Supportive Care and Survivorship: Managing Treatment Side Effects and Quality of Life Issues*

*Integrative Approaches to Breast Cancer Management: Nutrition, Exercise, and Mind-Body Therapies*

**ADVANCEMENTS IN BREAST CANCER RESEARCH**

## Health Economics of Breast Cancer: Cost-Effectiveness, Access to Care, and Health Policy Implications

## Patient Advocacy and Community Engagement: Empowering Patients and Promoting Awareness

## Future Directions in Breast Cancer Research: Emerging Technologies and Innovative Therapies

## CONCLUSION

**ADVANCEMENTS IN BREAST CANCER RESEARCH**

*Copyright © 2024 by Dr. Bernd Kortig*

*All Rights Reserved.*

*No part of this book may be used or reproduced by any means, graphic, electronic, or mechanical, including photocopying, recording, taping, or by any information storage retrieval system without the written permission of the Author.*

ADVANCEMENTS IN BREAST CANCER RESEARCH

# Introduction to Breast Cancer: Epidemiology, Incidence, and Mortality Trends

Breast cancer is a significant health concern worldwide, affecting millions of individuals each year. Understanding its epidemiology, incidence patterns, and mortality trends is crucial for public health planning, resource allocation, and developing effective prevention and control strategies.

Global Burden of Breast Cancer:

**ADVANCEMENTS IN BREAST CANCER RESEARCH**

Breast cancer is the most commonly diagnosed cancer among women globally, comprising approximately 25% of all female cancers. According to the World Health Organization (WHO), an estimated 2.3 million new cases of breast cancer were diagnosed worldwide in 2020, making it the leading cause of cancer-related morbidity and mortality among women.

Regional Variations:

The incidence of breast cancer varies widely by geographic region, with higher rates observed in developed countries compared to developing regions. For example, North America, Western Europe, and Australia have the highest age-standardized incidence rates, while rates are lower in Africa and parts of Asia. However, incidence rates in some developing countries are rising rapidly, reflecting changes in lifestyle, reproductive behaviors, and aging populations.

## ADVANCEMENTS IN BREAST CANCER RESEARCH

Trends Over Time:

Over the past few decades, there has been a notable increase in the incidence of breast cancer globally. This trend is attributed to several factors, including improvements in cancer detection and diagnosis, changes in reproductive patterns (e.g., delayed childbearing, fewer children), increased prevalence of obesity, adoption of Western lifestyles (e.g., sedentary behavior, high-fat diets), and environmental exposures (e.g., endocrine-disrupting chemicals).

Age-Specific Incidence:

Breast cancer incidence varies by age, with the majority of cases diagnosed in women aged 50 and older. However, breast cancer can occur at any age, and there is a notable increase in incidence among younger women in some populations. Early-onset breast cancer poses unique challenges in terms of

**ADVANCEMENTS IN BREAST CANCER RESEARCH**
diagnosis, treatment, and survivorship, underscoring the importance of targeted interventions for this age group.

Mortality Trends:

Despite advances in early detection and treatment, breast cancer remains a leading cause of cancer-related mortality among women worldwide. Mortality rates have declined in many high-income countries due to improvements in screening programs, access to effective therapies, and multidisciplinary care. However, mortality rates continue to rise in some low- and middle-income countries, highlighting disparities in healthcare access, quality of care, and socioeconomic factors.

Future Projections:

With aging populations and changing demographic trends, the global burden of

**ADVANCEMENTS IN BREAST CANCER RESEARCH**

breast cancer is expected to increase in the coming decades. Projections suggest that by 2040, the number of new breast cancer cases diagnosed annually could exceed 3 million worldwide, placing even greater strain on healthcare systems and resources.

**ADVANCEMENTS IN BREAST CANCER RESEARCH**

# Etiology and Risk Factors: Genetic, Environmental, and Lifestyle Influences

Breast cancer is a multifactorial disease with a complex etiology influenced by a combination of genetic, environmental, and lifestyle factors. Understanding these influences is crucial for identifying individuals at higher risk, implementing effective prevention strategies, and developing personalized approaches to screening and treatment.

Genetic Influences:

Genetic factors play a significant role in breast cancer risk, particularly in cases of hereditary breast cancer syndromes. The most well-known genes associated with hereditary breast cancer are

**ADVANCEMENTS IN BREAST CANCER RESEARCH**

BRCA1 and BRCA2. Mutations in these genes significantly increase the risk of developing both breast and ovarian cancers. However, mutations in other genes, such as TP53 (Li-Fraumeni syndrome), PTEN (Cowden syndrome), and PALB2, also contribute to an increased risk of breast cancer.

Family history is an essential component of genetic risk assessment. Individuals with a first-degree relative (parent, sibling, or child) diagnosed with breast cancer have a higher risk compared to the general population. Additionally, the age of onset of breast cancer in affected relatives and the presence of multiple affected family members can further increase the risk.

Environmental Influences:

Environmental factors encompass a wide range of exposures that can influence breast cancer risk. One well-established environmental risk factor is ionizing radiation. High-dose radiation exposure, such as that received during certain medical procedures or nuclear accidents, increases the risk of breast cancer development.

**ADVANCEMENTS IN BREAST CANCER RESEARCH**

Endocrine-disrupting chemicals (EDCs) found in various environmental contaminants, including pesticides, plastics, and industrial pollutants, have also been implicated in breast cancer etiology. EDCs can interfere with hormonal signaling pathways, potentially promoting tumor growth and progression.

Lifestyle Influences:

Lifestyle factors play a crucial role in breast cancer risk and prevention. Obesity is a significant risk factor for postmenopausal breast cancer, as adipose tissue serves as a source of estrogen production. Higher levels of estrogen in obese individuals can promote the growth of hormone receptor-positive breast cancers.

Physical activity has been consistently associated with a reduced risk of breast cancer. Regular exercise helps maintain a healthy weight and may also modulate hormone levels, immune function, and inflammation, all of which can impact breast cancer risk.

Alcohol consumption is another well-established lifestyle factor associated with breast cancer risk. Even moderate alcohol intake has been linked to an

**ADVANCEMENTS IN BREAST CANCER RESEARCH**

increased risk, with higher levels of consumption correlating with greater risk. Alcohol may influence breast cancer risk through various mechanisms, including alterations in hormone metabolism and DNA damage.

Dietary factors also play a role in breast cancer risk. A diet high in fruits, vegetables, whole grains, and lean protein sources is associated with a lower risk of breast cancer, while a diet high in processed meats, saturated fats, and sugary foods and beverages may increase the risk.

Interactions and Modifiers:

It's important to recognize that these genetic, environmental, and lifestyle factors do not act in isolation but often interact with one another to influence breast cancer risk. Additionally, individual characteristics such as age, reproductive history, hormonal factors, and socioeconomic status can modify the effects of these risk factors.

**ADVANCEMENTS IN BREAST CANCER RESEARCH**

# Biology of Breast Cancer: Oncogenes, Tumor Suppressor Genes, and Signaling Pathways

Breast cancer is a heterogeneous disease characterized by the dysregulation of multiple cellular processes, including cell growth, proliferation, differentiation, and survival. These aberrations often arise from genetic alterations that affect critical signaling pathways governing cellular behavior. Understanding the biology of breast cancer at the molecular level, including the role of oncogenes, tumor suppressor genes, and signaling pathways, is essential for elucidating disease mechanisms and developing targeted therapeutic strategies.

# ADVANCEMENTS IN BREAST CANCER RESEARCH

Oncogenes:

Oncogenes are genes that promote cell growth and proliferation when mutated or overexpressed. They encode proteins involved in signaling cascades that regulate key cellular processes. In breast cancer, several oncogenes have been identified as drivers of tumorigenesis, including:

1. HER2 (ERBB2): Amplification or overexpression of the human epidermal growth factor receptor 2 (HER2) gene is observed in approximately 20-25% of breast cancers. HER2 belongs to the epidermal growth factor receptor (EGFR) family and plays a crucial role in cell growth and survival signaling pathways. HER2-targeted therapies, such as trastuzumab and pertuzumab, have significantly improved outcomes for patients with HER2-positive breast cancer.
2. EGFR (ERBB1): The epidermal growth factor receptor (EGFR) is another member of the EGFR family implicated in breast cancer pathogenesis. EGFR overexpression is associated with aggressive tumor behavior and poor prognosis. Targeted therapies

**ADVANCEMENTS IN BREAST CANCER RESEARCH**

directed against EGFR, such as cetuximab and erlotinib, have been investigated in clinical trials, although their efficacy in breast cancer remains limited.

3. PIK3CA: Mutations in the phosphatidylinositol-4,5-bisphosphate 3-kinase catalytic subunit alpha (PIK3CA) gene are among the most common genetic alterations in breast cancer, occurring in approximately 30-40% of cases. PIK3CA encodes the catalytic subunit of phosphatidylinositol 3-kinase (PI3K), a key mediator of cell growth and survival signaling. Targeted inhibitors of the PI3K pathway, such as alpelisib and taselisib, have shown promise in clinical trials for PIK3CA-mutant breast cancer.

Tumor Suppressor Genes:

Tumor suppressor genes are genes that normally inhibit cell growth and division, acting as guardians of genomic integrity. Loss or inactivation of tumor suppressor genes contributes to unchecked cell proliferation and tumor development. Several tumor suppressor genes implicated in breast cancer include:

**ADVANCEMENTS IN BREAST CANCER RESEARCH**

1. TP53: The tumor protein p53 (TP53) gene is often referred to as the "guardian of the genome" due to its critical role in DNA repair, cell cycle regulation, and apoptosis. TP53 mutations are found in a significant proportion of breast cancers and are associated with aggressive tumor behavior and resistance to therapy.
2. BRCA1 and BRCA2: Mutations in the breast cancer susceptibility genes BRCA1 and BRCA2 predispose individuals to hereditary breast and ovarian cancer syndrome. These genes encode proteins involved in DNA repair mechanisms, and their loss of function leads to genomic instability and increased susceptibility to breast cancer development.
3. PTEN: Phosphatase and tensin homolog (PTEN) is a tumor suppressor gene that antagonizes the PI3K/AKT signaling pathway by dephosphorylating phosphatidylinositol 3,4,5-trisphosphate (PIP3). Loss of PTEN function results in hyperactivation of the PI3K pathway, promoting cell proliferation and survival.

Signaling Pathways:

**ADVANCEMENTS IN BREAST CANCER RESEARCH**

Several signaling pathways are dysregulated in breast cancer, driving tumor initiation, progression, and metastasis. Key signaling pathways implicated in breast cancer biology include:

1. PI3K/AKT/mTOR Pathway: The PI3K/AKT/mTOR pathway is a central signaling cascade involved in cell growth, proliferation, survival, and metabolism. Dysregulation of this pathway, often through mutations in PIK3CA or loss of PTEN function, is a common feature of breast cancer and represents a promising therapeutic target.
2. ER/PR Pathway: Estrogen receptor (ER) and progesterone receptor (PR) signaling pathways play crucial roles in the development and progression of hormone receptor-positive (HR+) breast cancers. These pathways regulate gene expression programs involved in cell proliferation, differentiation, and survival. Endocrine therapies targeting ER and PR, such as selective estrogen receptor modulators (SERMs) and aromatase inhibitors, are standard treatments for HR+ breast cancer.

**ADVANCEMENTS IN BREAST CANCER RESEARCH**

3. MAPK/ERK Pathway: The mitogen-activated protein kinase (MAPK)/extracellular signal-regulated kinase (ERK) pathway is activated downstream of receptor tyrosine kinases (RTKs), such as EGFR and HER2. Dysregulated MAPK/ERK signaling promotes cell proliferation, survival, and metastasis in breast cancer, highlighting its importance as a therapeutic target.

ADVANCEMENTS IN BREAST CANCER RESEARCH

# Breast Anatomy and Physiology: Normal Development and Function

The human breast is a complex organ composed of glandular tissue, ducts, adipose tissue, and supportive structures. Its primary function is to produce milk for nourishing offspring, but it also serves important roles in sexual attraction, maternal bonding, and overall body aesthetics. Understanding the normal anatomy and physiology of the breast is essential for appreciating its development, function, and potential pathologies.

Anatomy of the Breast:

The breast is located on the anterior chest wall, spanning from the second to the sixth rib and extending from the sternum to the axilla (armpit). Each breast is comprised of 15-20 lobes arranged in a radial pattern around the nipple. Within each lobe are numerous lobules, which contain clusters of milk-producing alveoli. These lobules are connected to ducts that converge toward the nipple, where milk is released during lactation.

The breast is supported by ligaments called Cooper's ligaments, which attach the glandular tissue to the overlying skin and underlying chest wall. Adipose tissue surrounds the glandular tissue and provides cushioning and insulation. Blood vessels, lymphatic vessels, and nerves supply and innervate the breast, facilitating its physiological functions.

Development of the Breast:

Breast development begins during embryogenesis and continues through puberty, pregnancy, and lactation. In females, the rudimentary mammary glands develop from the ectoderm along the mammary ridges (milk lines), which extend from the axilla to the groin. During fetal development, these mammary ridges regress except for the two regions overlying the pectoral muscles, where the breasts will eventually form.

At puberty, hormonal changes, particularly estrogen and progesterone, stimulate further development of

**ADVANCEMENTS IN BREAST CANCER RESEARCH**

the breast tissue. This results in the growth of ductal and glandular tissue, accompanied by increased vascularity and adipose deposition. The areola, the pigmented area surrounding the nipple, also enlarges and becomes more prominent.

Physiology of the Breast:

The primary physiological function of the breast is lactation, which supports infant nutrition and immunological protection. Milk production is regulated by a complex interplay of hormones and neuroendocrine signals. During pregnancy, rising levels of estrogen, progesterone, and prolactin stimulate the growth and differentiation of mammary alveoli in preparation for lactation.

Following childbirth, the release of placental hormones triggers milk production (lactogenesis). Prolactin, secreted by the anterior pituitary gland, stimulates milk synthesis in the mammary alveoli, while oxytocin, released from the posterior pituitary gland, promotes milk ejection (let-down reflex) by causing contraction of the myoepithelial cells surrounding the alveoli.

Breast milk is a complex fluid containing a balanced combination of macronutrients (e.g., carbohydrates,

**ADVANCEMENTS IN BREAST CANCER RESEARCH**

proteins, fats), micronutrients (e.g., vitamins, minerals), bioactive compounds (e.g., antibodies, enzymes, growth factors), and immune cells (e.g., leukocytes). It provides essential nutrients for infant growth and development, confers passive immunity against infections, and promotes maternal-infant bonding.

In addition to lactation, the breast also undergoes cyclical changes during the menstrual cycle in response to hormonal fluctuations. These changes, including breast swelling, tenderness, and nodularity, are influenced by estrogen and progesterone levels and typically peak during the premenstrual phase.

ADVANCEMENTS IN BREAST CANCER RESEARCH

# Pathology of Breast Cancer: Histological Subtypes and Molecular Classification

Breast cancer is a heterogeneous disease with diverse histological subtypes and molecular profiles, each with distinct clinicopathological characteristics and therapeutic implications. Pathological evaluation plays a crucial role in diagnosing breast cancer, determining prognosis, and guiding treatment decisions. Understanding the histological subtypes and molecular classification of breast cancer is essential for accurate diagnosis and personalized management strategies.

Histological Subtypes:

**ADVANCEMENTS IN BREAST CANCER RESEARCH**

1. Invasive Ductal Carcinoma (IDC): IDC is the most common histological subtype of breast cancer, accounting for approximately 70-80% of cases. It arises from the epithelial cells lining the milk ducts and typically presents as irregular, infiltrating tumor masses with glandular or ductal architecture on histological examination.
2. Invasive Lobular Carcinoma (ILC): ILC accounts for 5-15% of breast cancers and originates from the lobules or terminal ductal-lobular units. Unlike IDC, ILC tends to infiltrate the breast tissue in a single-file pattern, making it less conspicuous on imaging studies. Histologically, ILC is characterized by small, discohesive cells with minimal glandular formation.
3. Ductal Carcinoma In Situ (DCIS): DCIS is a non-invasive form of breast cancer in which malignant cells are confined to the ductal epithelium without invading the surrounding stroma. Although DCIS is not invasive, it has the potential to progress to invasive carcinoma if left untreated. Histologically, DCIS lesions exhibit varying degrees of architectural complexity and cytological atypia.

**ADVANCEMENTS IN BREAST CANCER RESEARCH**

4. Lobular Carcinoma In Situ (LCIS): LCIS is a non-obligate precursor lesion characterized by the proliferation of abnormal cells within the lobules. Unlike DCIS, LCIS does not exhibit architectural distortion or cytological atypia and is considered a marker of increased breast cancer risk rather than a direct precursor to invasive disease.
5. Special Histological Subtypes: Breast cancer can also present with special histological subtypes, such as mucinous (colloid), papillary, medullary, metaplastic, and tubular carcinomas. These subtypes have distinct morphological features and may carry prognostic significance.

Molecular Classification:

Advances in molecular biology have led to the identification of distinct molecular subtypes of breast cancer based on gene expression profiling and molecular markers. The most widely used classification system is the intrinsic molecular subtyping proposed by Perou et al., which categorizes breast cancer into four main subtypes:

**ADVANCEMENTS IN BREAST CANCER RESEARCH**

1. Luminal A: Luminal A tumors are characterized by the expression of estrogen receptor (ER) and/or progesterone receptor (PR) and low proliferative activity (low Ki-67). They typically have a favorable prognosis and are sensitive to endocrine therapies such as tamoxifen or aromatase inhibitors.
2. Luminal B: Luminal B tumors also express ER and/or PR but have higher proliferative activity (high Ki-67) and may exhibit HER2 overexpression or amplification. Luminal B tumors tend to have a poorer prognosis compared to Luminal A tumors and may require more aggressive treatment approaches.
3. HER2-enriched: HER2-enriched tumors overexpress the human epidermal growth factor receptor 2 (HER2) protein due to gene amplification. They are typically ER and PR negative and have high proliferative activity. HER2-enriched tumors are associated with aggressive tumor behavior but are highly responsive to HER2-targeted therapies such as trastuzumab and pertuzumab.
4. Triple-negative Breast Cancer (TNBC): TNBC is characterized by the absence of ER, PR, and HER2 expression. TNBC tumors are heterogeneous and exhibit high

## ADVANCEMENTS IN BREAST CANCER RESEARCH

proliferative activity. They are associated with a poorer prognosis and limited treatment options compared to other subtypes.

In addition to the intrinsic molecular subtypes, breast cancer can be classified based on specific molecular alterations, such as mutations in the BRCA1/2 genes, PIK3CA mutations, and gene expression signatures related to proliferation, immune response, and stromal interactions.

ADVANCEMENTS IN BREAST CANCER RESEARCH

# Early Detection and Screening Strategies: Mammography, MRI, Ultrasound, and Biomarkers

Early detection of breast cancer plays a crucial role in improving prognosis and reducing mortality rates. Screening strategies aim to identify breast cancer at an early stage when treatment is more effective and less invasive. Mammography, magnetic resonance imaging (MRI), ultrasound, and biomarkers are important tools utilized in breast cancer screening and early detection efforts. Each modality has its advantages, limitations, and recommended indications, contributing to a

**ADVANCEMENTS IN BREAST CANCER RESEARCH**
comprehensive approach to breast cancer screening.

Mammography:

Mammography is the most widely used and established screening tool for breast cancer. It involves obtaining X-ray images of the breast tissue, typically in two views (mediolateral oblique and craniocaudal), to detect abnormalities such as masses, microcalcifications, and architectural distortions. Mammography has demonstrated efficacy in reducing breast cancer mortality through early detection, particularly in women aged 50 and older.

Advantages of mammography include:

1. High sensitivity for detecting breast cancer, especially in women with dense breast tissue.
2. Wide availability and established infrastructure for screening programs.
3. Cost-effectiveness compared to other imaging modalities.

## ADVANCEMENTS IN BREAST CANCER RESEARCH

Limitations of mammography include:

1. Reduced sensitivity in women with dense breast tissue, which may obscure small lesions.
2. False-positive findings leading to unnecessary follow-up tests and anxiety.
3. Limited sensitivity for detecting certain types of breast cancer, such as lobular carcinoma and in situ lesions.

MRI (Magnetic Resonance Imaging):

MRI is a highly sensitive imaging modality that uses magnetic fields and radio waves to generate detailed images of the breast tissue. It is recommended as an adjunctive screening tool for women at high risk of developing breast cancer, such as those with a strong family history or carriers of BRCA1/2 mutations. MRI is particularly useful in detecting invasive lobular carcinoma and evaluating the extent of disease in women with dense breast tissue or a history of prior breast cancer.

Advantages of MRI include:

**ADVANCEMENTS IN BREAST CANCER RESEARCH**
1. High sensitivity for detecting small and invasive cancers, especially in high-risk populations.
2. Multiplanar imaging capability, providing comprehensive assessment of breast morphology and vascularity.
3. Ability to detect occult lesions not visualized on mammography or ultrasound.

Limitations of MRI include:

1. Lower specificity compared to mammography, leading to higher rates of false-positive findings and unnecessary biopsies.
2. Cost and resource-intensive nature of MRI examinations.
3. Limited availability and expertise in interpretation, particularly in community settings.

Ultrasound:

Ultrasound utilizes sound waves to produce real-time images of the breast tissue and is often

## ADVANCEMENTS IN BREAST CANCER RESEARCH

used as a supplemental imaging modality in breast cancer screening. It is particularly useful in characterizing breast masses detected on mammography or MRI, differentiating between solid and cystic lesions, and guiding needle biopsies. Ultrasound is also valuable in evaluating young women and women with dense breast tissue, where mammography may be less sensitive.

Advantages of ultrasound include:

1. No radiation exposure, making it safe for repeated examinations, including during pregnancy and lactation.
2. Dynamic real-time imaging, allowing for accurate characterization of lesions and guidance for interventional procedures.
3. High sensitivity for detecting cysts, solid masses, and axillary lymph nodes.

Limitations of ultrasound include:

1. Operator-dependent technique, with variability in image quality and interpretation.

**ADVANCEMENTS IN BREAST CANCER RESEARCH**

2. Limited ability to detect microcalcifications and ductal carcinoma in situ (DCIS).
3. Difficulty in distinguishing between benign and malignant lesions, leading to increased rates of false-positive findings and unnecessary biopsies.

Biomarkers:

Biomarkers are molecular or genetic markers that can be measured in blood, tissue, or other bodily fluids and used to assess an individual's risk of developing breast cancer or to aid in early detection and prognosis. Several biomarkers have been identified as potential tools for breast cancer screening and risk assessment, including:

1. Breast Density: Breast density, determined by mammographic imaging, is an established risk factor for breast cancer. Women with dense breast tissue have a higher risk of developing breast cancer and may benefit from supplemental screening modalities such as MRI or ultrasound.
2. Genetic Mutations: Genetic mutations, such as mutations in the BRCA1/2 genes, are

associated with an increased risk of developing breast cancer. Genetic testing and counseling can identify individuals with hereditary breast cancer syndromes who may benefit from enhanced surveillance and risk-reducing strategies.

3. Serum Biomarkers: Several serum biomarkers, such as carcinoembryonic antigen (CEA), cancer antigen 15-3 (CA 15-3), and carbohydrate antigen 27.29 (CA 27.29), have been investigated as potential tools for breast cancer screening and monitoring. However, their utility in routine clinical practice remains limited due to issues related to sensitivity, specificity, and standardization.

4. Molecular Profiling: Gene expression profiling assays, such as Oncotype DX, MammaPrint, and Prosigna, provide valuable information about the molecular subtype, aggressiveness, and prognosis of breast cancer. These assays can aid in treatment decision-making, particularly in hormone receptor-positive breast cancer, by predicting the likelihood of recurrence and guiding the use of adjuvant therapies.

**ADVANCEMENTS IN BREAST CANCER RESEARCH**

# Tumor Microenvironment: Role of Stromal Cells, Immune Cells, and Extracellular Matrix

The tumor microenvironment (TME) is a dynamic and complex ecosystem consisting of cancer cells, stromal cells, immune cells, blood vessels, and extracellular matrix (ECM) components. Interactions within the TME play a critical role in tumor initiation, progression, metastasis, and response to therapy. Understanding the cellular and molecular components of the TME and their functional contributions is essential for developing effective cancer treatments and improving patient outcomes.

Stromal Cells:

**ADVANCEMENTS IN BREAST CANCER RESEARCH**

1. Cancer-Associated Fibroblasts (CAFs): CAFs are one of the most abundant stromal cell types in the TME and play a crucial role in tumor progression. They promote tumor growth, invasion, angiogenesis, and metastasis through the secretion of growth factors, cytokines, and ECM-modifying enzymes. CAFs also remodel the ECM, creating a supportive niche for cancer cell survival and dissemination.
2. Endothelial Cells: Endothelial cells form the inner lining of blood vessels and play a central role in tumor angiogenesis, the process by which new blood vessels are formed to supply nutrients and oxygen to the growing tumor. Tumor-associated endothelial cells exhibit abnormal morphology and function, contributing to tumor vascularization and facilitating tumor cell intravasation and metastasis.
3. Pericytes: Pericytes are mural cells that wrap around blood vessels and regulate vascular stability and function. In the TME, pericytes interact with endothelial cells to maintain vascular integrity and modulate angiogenic signaling pathways. Dysregulated pericyte function can lead to abnormal vessel

formation, leakiness, and increased tumor aggressiveness.

Immune Cells:

1. Tumor-Infiltrating Lymphocytes (TILs): TILs are immune cells that infiltrate the tumor tissue and play a critical role in anti-tumor immunity. TILs include cytotoxic T cells, which can directly kill cancer cells, as well as helper T cells, regulatory T cells, and natural killer (NK) cells, which regulate immune responses within the TME. High levels of TILs are associated with improved prognosis and response to immunotherapy in some cancer types.
2. Tumor-Associated Macrophages (TAMs): TAMs are a heterogeneous population of macrophages that are recruited to the TME by tumor-derived chemokines and cytokines. Depending on their polarization state, TAMs can exert pro-tumorigenic (M2-like) or anti-tumorigenic (M1-like) effects. M2-like TAMs promote tumor growth, angiogenesis, and immunosuppression, whereas M1-like

TAMs facilitate tumor regression and anti-tumor immune responses.
3. Myeloid-Derived Suppressor Cells (MDSCs): MDSCs are a population of immature myeloid cells with potent immunosuppressive activity. In the TME, MDSCs inhibit anti-tumor immune responses by suppressing the function of T cells, NK cells, and dendritic cells. MDSCs also promote tumor progression by facilitating angiogenesis, metastasis, and immune evasion.

Extracellular Matrix (ECM):

The ECM is a complex network of proteins, glycoproteins, and proteoglycans that provide structural support and regulate cellular behavior within the TME. Key ECM components include collagen, fibronectin, laminin, and hyaluronic acid. In addition to its structural role, the ECM acts as a reservoir for growth factors and cytokines, modulates cell adhesion, migration, and invasion, and influences tumor-stromal interactions.

**ADVANCEMENTS IN BREAST CANCER RESEARCH**

1. Remodeling and Stiffening: Tumor-associated ECM undergoes extensive remodeling and stiffening, driven by increased deposition of collagen and other ECM components by CAFs and tumor cells. ECM stiffness promotes tumor progression by enhancing cancer cell survival, proliferation, invasion, and metastasis, as well as by modulating immune cell function and drug resistance.
2. Cell-ECM Interactions: Cell-ECM interactions play a critical role in tumor cell behavior and phenotype. Integrin-mediated adhesion to the ECM regulates cell proliferation, survival, and migration, while ECM-derived signals modulate intracellular signaling pathways involved in tumorigenesis and metastasis. Disruption of cell-ECM interactions can impair tumor cell invasion and metastasis, making it an attractive target for cancer therapy.
3. Angiogenesis and Vascularization: The ECM provides a scaffold for new blood vessel formation and guides endothelial cell migration and tube formation during angiogenesis. ECM-derived signaling molecules, such as vascular endothelial growth factor (VEGF), fibroblast growth

**ADVANCEMENTS IN BREAST CANCER RESEARCH**

factor (FGF), and matrix metalloproteinases (MMPs), regulate angiogenic processes within the TME, facilitating tumor vascularization and metastasis.

ADVANCEMENTS IN BREAST CANCER RESEARCH

# Metastasis: Mechanisms, Key Players, and Therapeutic Targets

Metastasis is the process by which cancer cells spread from the primary tumor site to distant organs or tissues, where they establish secondary tumors. Metastasis is a complex and multistep process involving a series of sequential events that enable cancer cells to invade surrounding tissues, intravasate into blood or lymphatic vessels, survive in circulation, extravasate at distant sites, and colonize new microenvironments. Understanding the mechanisms of metastasis, identifying key players involved, and targeting critical pathways represent important areas of research for developing effective cancer therapies and improving patient outcomes.

Mechanisms of Metastasis:

**ADVANCEMENTS IN BREAST CANCER RESEARCH**

1. Invasion: Cancer cells acquire invasive properties through a process known as epithelial-mesenchymal transition (EMT), which involves the loss of epithelial characteristics and the acquisition of mesenchymal features. EMT allows cancer cells to detach from the primary tumor mass, invade surrounding tissues, and penetrate the basement membrane, facilitating their entry into blood or lymphatic vessels.
2. Intravasation: Once cancer cells have invaded surrounding tissues, they may enter nearby blood or lymphatic vessels through a process called intravasation. Intravasation involves interactions between cancer cells and endothelial cells lining the vessel walls, allowing cancer cells to penetrate the vessel barrier and enter the circulation.
3. Survival in Circulation: Cancer cells face numerous challenges in the bloodstream, including shear stress, immune surveillance, and anoikis (detachment-induced cell death). To survive in circulation, cancer cells may form clusters, interact with platelets or leukocytes, and undergo phenotypic changes to evade immune detection and anoikis.

## ADVANCEMENTS IN BREAST CANCER RESEARCH

4. Extravasation: Upon reaching distant organs or tissues, cancer cells must extravasate from the circulation to establish secondary tumors. Extravasation involves adhesion to endothelial cells, transmigration across the vessel wall, and interaction with the local microenvironment at the secondary site.
5. Colonization: Once cancer cells have extravasated into the parenchyma of distant organs, they must adapt to the new microenvironment and initiate tumor growth. Colonization involves interactions with stromal cells, remodeling of the extracellular matrix, and establishment of a supportive niche for tumor cell survival and proliferation.

Key Players in Metastasis:

1. Tumor Microenvironment: The tumor microenvironment plays a critical role in modulating metastatic behavior. Stromal cells, including cancer-associated fibroblasts, endothelial cells, and immune cells, contribute to the formation of a supportive niche for metastatic colonization. Extracellular matrix components, such as

collagen, fibronectin, and hyaluronic acid, provide structural support and signaling cues that promote metastatic progression.
2. Epithelial-Mesenchymal Transition (EMT): EMT is a key cellular program that confers invasive and migratory properties to cancer cells during metastasis. Transcription factors such as Snail, Slug, Twist, and Zeb1/2 orchestrate the EMT process by repressing epithelial genes and activating mesenchymal genes, leading to changes in cell morphology, motility, and invasiveness.
3. Angiogenesis and Lymphangiogenesis: Angiogenesis, the formation of new blood vessels, and lymphangiogenesis, the formation of new lymphatic vessels, play crucial roles in facilitating tumor metastasis. Angiogenic factors such as vascular endothelial growth factor (VEGF) promote the sprouting of blood vessels from existing vasculature, providing a route for cancer cell dissemination. Lymphangiogenic factors such as VEGF-C and VEGF-D similarly promote lymphatic vessel growth and metastatic spread via the lymphatic system.
4. Extracellular Matrix Remodeling: Cancer cells modify the extracellular matrix (ECM) of the primary tumor and distant organs to

## ADVANCEMENTS IN BREAST CANCER RESEARCH

facilitate metastasis. Matrix metalloproteinases (MMPs) and other proteases degrade ECM components, allowing cancer cells to penetrate tissue barriers and invade surrounding tissues. ECM proteins such as fibronectin and laminin provide adhesive substrates for cancer cell migration and invasion.

Therapeutic Targets in Metastasis:

1. Targeting EMT: Inhibiting key regulators of EMT, such as transcription factors (e.g., Snail, Twist) or signaling pathways (e.g., TGF-β, Wnt), represents a potential strategy for blocking the invasive and migratory properties of cancer cells.
2. Anti-Angiogenic Therapy: Targeting angiogenesis with inhibitors of VEGF or other pro-angiogenic factors can disrupt tumor vascularization and inhibit metastatic spread by depriving tumors of oxygen and nutrients.
3. Inhibition of Extracellular Matrix Remodeling: MMP inhibitors and other agents targeting ECM remodeling enzymes may prevent

**ADVANCEMENTS IN BREAST CANCER RESEARCH**

cancer cell invasion and metastasis by stabilizing tissue barriers and blocking ECM degradation.

4. Immune Checkpoint Inhibition: Immune checkpoint inhibitors, such as anti-PD-1/PD-L1 antibodies, can enhance anti-tumor immune responses and inhibit metastatic progression by activating cytotoxic T cells and overcoming immune evasion mechanisms within the TME.
5. Targeting Metastatic Niches: Disrupting the supportive microenvironment at metastatic sites, either through inhibition of stromal cell interactions.

**ADVANCEMENTS IN BREAST CANCER RESEARCH**

# Animal Models

Animal models play a crucial role in breast cancer research and drug development by recapitulating key aspects of human breast cancer biology, progression, and response to therapy. These models provide valuable tools for investigating disease mechanisms, evaluating novel therapeutic agents, and predicting clinical outcomes. In this comprehensive overview, we will explore the utility of various animal models of breast cancer and their contributions to advancing our understanding of the disease and improving patient care.

Types of Animal Models:

1. Mouse Models: Mice are the most commonly used species for modeling breast cancer due to their genetic, physiological, and immunological similarities to humans. Genetically engineered mouse models (GEMMs) can be engineered to develop

spontaneous mammary tumors by altering the expression of oncogenes (e.g., HER2, MYC) or tumor suppressor genes (e.g., TP53, BRCA1/2). Additionally, patient-derived xenograft (PDX) models involve the transplantation of human breast cancer cells or tissues into immunocompromised mice to study tumor growth, metastasis, and therapeutic responses.

2. Rat Models: Rat models of breast cancer offer advantages such as larger size, longer lifespan, and a closer resemblance to human breast anatomy and physiology compared to mice. Chemically-induced mammary carcinogenesis models, such as the 7,12-dimethylbenz[a]anthracene (DMBA) or N-methyl-N-nitrosourea (MNU) models, involve the administration of carcinogens to induce mammary tumors in rats. These models are valuable for studying tumor initiation, progression, and chemoprevention strategies.

3. Canine Models: Dogs naturally develop mammary tumors that share histological and molecular similarities with human breast cancer. Canine mammary tumor models provide an opportunity to study spontaneous

**ADVANCEMENTS IN BREAST CANCER RESEARCH**

tumor development in a large animal species with an intact immune system. These models offer insights into tumor biology, metastasis, and therapeutic responses, as well as potential translational implications for both veterinary and human medicine.

Utility in Research:

1. Disease Mechanisms: Animal models of breast cancer facilitate the study of disease mechanisms underlying tumor initiation, progression, metastasis, and therapy resistance. By manipulating genetic or environmental factors, researchers can elucidate the roles of specific genes, signaling pathways, and microenvironmental interactions in breast cancer pathogenesis.
2. Preclinical Drug Testing: Animal models serve as valuable preclinical platforms for evaluating the efficacy, safety, and pharmacokinetics of investigational drugs and therapeutic interventions. These models allow researchers to assess tumor response to conventional chemotherapy, targeted therapies, immunotherapies, and

experimental agents in vivo before clinical trials in human patients.
3. Biomarker Discovery: Animal models enable the identification and validation of biomarkers associated with breast cancer prognosis, treatment response, and disease recurrence. By analyzing tumor tissues, blood samples, and imaging data from animal studies, researchers can identify candidate biomarkers for further validation in clinical settings.

Drug Development:

1. Target Identification and Validation: Animal models help identify potential therapeutic targets and validate their relevance in breast cancer biology. By manipulating gene expression or pharmacological targeting in animal models, researchers can assess the effects on tumor growth, metastasis, and survival, providing evidence for target prioritization in drug development.
2. Drug Screening and Optimization: Animal models serve as invaluable tools for screening and optimizing novel therapeutic

agents for breast cancer treatment. By testing drug candidates in vivo, researchers can evaluate their efficacy, toxicity, and pharmacokinetic profiles, guiding dose selection, formulation optimization, and combination therapy strategies.
3. Translational Relevance: Findings from animal studies can inform the design and implementation of clinical trials in human patients, leading to the development of new treatment modalities and personalized therapeutic approaches. Animal models provide essential preclinical data to support regulatory approval and clinical translation of novel drugs and therapeutic interventions.

Challenges and Considerations:

1. Relevance to Human Disease: Despite their utility, animal models may not fully recapitulate the complexity and heterogeneity of human breast cancer. Variations in tumor biology, microenvironmental interactions, and immune responses between species can

limit the translational relevance of preclinical findings.
2. Ethical and Welfare Considerations: The use of animals in research raises ethical and welfare considerations, necessitating adherence to rigorous standards of animal care, welfare, and ethical oversight. Researchers must prioritize the principles of the 3Rs (Replacement, Reduction, Refinement) to minimize animal suffering and ensure scientific rigor.
3. Translational Challenges: Translating preclinical findings from animal models to clinical practice poses challenges related to species differences, predictive validity, and therapeutic response heterogeneity. Close collaboration between basic researchers, clinicians, and regulatory agencies is essential for addressing these challenges and maximizing the translational impact of preclinical research.

ADVANCEMENTS IN BREAST CANCER RESEARCH

# Imaging Techniques in Breast Cancer Diagnosis and Monitoring

Imaging techniques play a crucial role in the diagnosis, staging, treatment planning, and monitoring of breast cancer. These techniques allow for non-invasive visualization of breast tissue, detection of abnormalities, characterization of tumors, and assessment of treatment response. In this comprehensive overview, we will discuss the various imaging modalities used in breast cancer diagnosis and monitoring, including mammography, ultrasound, magnetic resonance imaging (MRI), molecular imaging, and emerging technologies.

1. Mammography:

Mammography is the gold standard imaging modality for breast cancer screening and diagnosis. It involves obtaining low-dose X-ray images of the

**ADVANCEMENTS IN BREAST CANCER RESEARCH**

breast tissue to detect abnormalities such as masses, microcalcifications, and architectural distortions. Digital mammography has largely replaced traditional film-screen mammography due to its superior image quality, faster image acquisition, and ease of image manipulation. Mammography is particularly effective in detecting early-stage breast cancer in asymptomatic women and remains the cornerstone of population-based screening programs.

2. Ultrasound:

Ultrasound imaging utilizes high-frequency sound waves to produce real-time images of the breast tissue. It is commonly used as a supplemental imaging modality to evaluate breast abnormalities detected on mammography or clinical examination, characterize breast masses, and guide interventional procedures such as biopsies and cyst aspirations. Ultrasound is particularly valuable in differentiating between solid and cystic lesions, evaluating axillary lymph nodes, and assessing breast density, especially in women with dense breast tissue.

3. Magnetic Resonance Imaging (MRI):

**ADVANCEMENTS IN BREAST CANCER RESEARCH**
Breast MRI is a powerful imaging modality that provides detailed anatomical and functional information about breast tissue. It uses magnetic fields and radio waves to generate high-resolution images of the breast, including dynamic contrast-enhanced (DCE) sequences that assess tissue vascularity and diffusion-weighted imaging (DWI) sequences that evaluate tissue cellularity. Breast MRI is indicated for screening high-risk individuals, evaluating extent of disease in newly diagnosed breast cancer patients, assessing response to neoadjuvant chemotherapy, and detecting recurrent or residual disease after treatment.

4. Molecular Imaging:

Molecular imaging techniques such as positron emission tomography (PET) and single-photon emission computed tomography (SPECT) enable non-invasive visualization of biological processes at the molecular and cellular level. PET imaging with radiotracers such as fluorodeoxyglucose (FDG) can assess tumor metabolism and detect distant metastases in breast cancer patients. Other molecular imaging approaches, such as optical imaging and molecular MRI, utilize targeted contrast agents to visualize specific biomarkers or

**ADVANCEMENTS IN BREAST CANCER RESEARCH**
molecular pathways associated with breast cancer progression and response to therapy.

5. Emerging Technologies:

Recent advancements in imaging technology have led to the development of novel techniques for breast cancer diagnosis and monitoring. These include:

- Contrast-Enhanced Mammography (CEM): CEM combines conventional mammography with intravenous contrast administration to improve the detection and characterization of breast lesions, particularly in women with dense breast tissue or indeterminate findings on conventional mammography.
- Tomosynthesis: Digital breast tomosynthesis (DBT) is an advanced form of mammography that generates 3D images of the breast tissue, reducing the overlapping of structures and improving lesion detection and characterization compared to traditional 2D mammography.
- Ultrasound Elastography: Elastography measures tissue stiffness or elasticity and can help differentiate between benign and

## ADVANCEMENTS IN BREAST CANCER RESEARCH

malignant breast lesions based on their mechanical properties. It is often used as a supplemental imaging technique to conventional ultrasound for lesion characterization.
- Artificial Intelligence (AI): AI-driven imaging algorithms and computer-aided detection (CAD) systems are being developed to assist radiologists in interpreting breast imaging studies, improving accuracy, efficiency, and diagnostic confidence in breast cancer diagnosis and monitoring.

Clinical Applications:

Imaging techniques play a critical role in various aspects of breast cancer care, including:

- Screening and Early Detection: Mammography screening programs have been shown to reduce breast cancer mortality by detecting tumors at an early stage when treatment is most effective. Emerging technologies such as CEM and DBT offer improved sensitivity and specificity

for lesion detection, particularly in women with dense breast tissue.
- Diagnosis and Staging: Imaging modalities such as ultrasound, MRI, and PET/CT are used to evaluate breast abnormalities detected on clinical examination or screening mammography, determine tumor extent and involvement of regional lymph nodes, and stage breast cancer prior to treatment initiation.
- Treatment Planning: Imaging studies play a crucial role in treatment planning and decision-making, guiding the selection of appropriate surgical, radiation, and systemic therapy options based on tumor size, location, biology, and extent of disease.
- Response Assessment: During and after treatment, imaging techniques such as MRI, ultrasound, and PET/CT are used to assess treatment response, monitor tumor regression or progression, and detect residual or recurrent disease.
- Surveillance and Follow-Up: Following completion of primary treatment, imaging surveillance with mammography, ultrasound, or MRI is performed at regular intervals to monitor for disease recurrence, assess

**ADVANCEMENTS IN BREAST CANCER RESEARCH**
treatment efficacy, and ensure long-term disease-free survival.

ADVANCEMENTS IN BREAST CANCER RESEARCH

# Biomarkers in Breast Cancer: Prognostic, Predictive, and Therapeutic Targets

Breast cancer is a heterogeneous disease with diverse molecular subtypes, clinical behaviors, and treatment responses. Prognostic, predictive, and therapeutic targets play critical roles in guiding treatment decisions, predicting patient outcomes, and developing targeted therapies for breast cancer. In this comprehensive overview, we will discuss the significance of prognostic and predictive factors, as well as therapeutic targets, in breast cancer management.

**ADVANCEMENTS IN BREAST CANCER RESEARCH**
1. Prognostic Factors:

Prognostic factors provide information about the likelihood of disease recurrence, metastasis, and overall survival independent of treatment. These factors help stratify patients into risk categories and inform treatment decisions. Common prognostic factors in breast cancer include:

- Tumor Size and Stage: Tumor size and extent of spread to regional lymph nodes and distant organs (stage) are strong prognostic indicators in breast cancer. Larger tumor size and advanced stage are associated with poorer outcomes and higher risk of recurrence.
- Histological Grade: Histological grade reflects the degree of tumor differentiation and aggressiveness. High-grade tumors with poorly differentiated cells tend to be more aggressive and have a worse prognosis compared to low-grade tumors.

**ADVANCEMENTS IN BREAST CANCER RESEARCH**

- Lymph Node Involvement: The presence of metastasis in axillary lymph nodes is a strong prognostic factor in breast cancer. Patients with positive lymph nodes have a higher risk of disease recurrence and poorer survival outcomes compared to those with negative lymph nodes.
- Hormone Receptor Status: Estrogen receptor (ER), progesterone receptor (PR), and human epidermal growth factor receptor 2 (HER2) status are important prognostic factors in breast cancer. Hormone receptor-positive tumors tend to have a more favorable prognosis than hormone receptor-negative tumors, while HER2-positive tumors are associated with a higher risk of recurrence.
- Ki-67 Proliferation Index: Ki-67 is a marker of cellular proliferation, and high Ki-67 expression is associated with more aggressive tumor behavior and poorer prognosis in breast cancer.
- Molecular Subtypes: Breast cancer can be classified into different molecular subtypes based on gene expression profiles, including luminal A, luminal B, HER2-enriched, and triple-negative/basal-like subtypes. Molecular subtyping provides valuable prognostic

**ADVANCEMENTS IN BREAST CANCER RESEARCH**
information and helps guide treatment decisions.

2. Predictive Factors:

Predictive factors are biomarkers that predict the likelihood of response to specific therapies and guide treatment selection. Identifying predictive factors allows for personalized treatment approaches tailored to individual patient characteristics. Common predictive factors in breast cancer include:

- Hormone Receptor Status: Hormone receptor-positive tumors are sensitive to endocrine therapies such as tamoxifen, aromatase inhibitors, and selective estrogen receptor modulators (SERMs). Patients with hormone receptor-positive disease are more likely to benefit from endocrine therapy compared to those with hormone receptor-negative disease.

**ADVANCEMENTS IN BREAST CANCER RESEARCH**

- HER2 Status: HER2-positive breast cancers overexpress the HER2/neu oncogene and are sensitive to HER2-targeted therapies such as trastuzumab, pertuzumab, and ado-trastuzumab emtansine (T-DM1). HER2-positive patients derive significant benefit from HER2-targeted therapy in combination with chemotherapy.
- BRCA Mutation Status: Breast cancer patients with germline mutations in the BRCA1 or BRCA2 genes are more likely to respond to platinum-based chemotherapy and PARP inhibitors such as olaparib and talazoparib. BRCA mutation status guides treatment decisions and eligibility for targeted therapies.
- PD-L1 Expression: Programmed death-ligand 1 (PD-L1) expression in tumor-infiltrating immune cells is a predictive biomarker for response to immune checkpoint inhibitors such as pembrolizumab and atezolizumab in metastatic triple-negative breast cancer.
- Genomic Profiling: Gene expression profiling assays, such as Oncotype DX, MammaPrint, and Prosigna, provide predictive information about the likelihood of recurrence and response to chemotherapy or endocrine

**ADVANCEMENTS IN BREAST CANCER RESEARCH**

therapy. Genomic profiling helps identify patients who may benefit from adjuvant chemotherapy or hormonal therapy.

3. Therapeutic Targets:

Therapeutic targets are molecular entities that can be targeted by drugs or therapeutic interventions to inhibit tumor growth, metastasis, and survival. Targeted therapies aim to exploit specific molecular aberrations or vulnerabilities in cancer cells while sparing normal tissues. Common therapeutic targets in breast cancer include:

- Hormone Receptors: Estrogen receptor (ER) and progesterone receptor (PR) are targets for endocrine therapies such as tamoxifen, aromatase inhibitors, and fulvestrant. Targeting hormone receptors blocks estrogen signaling and inhibits tumor growth in hormone receptor-positive breast cancer.

**ADVANCEMENTS IN BREAST CANCER RESEARCH**
- Human Epidermal Growth Factor Receptor 2 (HER2): HER2-targeted therapies, including monoclonal antibodies (trastuzumab, pertuzumab), antibody-drug conjugates (T-DM1), and tyrosine kinase inhibitors (lapatinib, neratinib), inhibit HER2 signaling and improve outcomes in HER2-positive breast.

**ADVANCEMENTS IN BREAST CANCER RESEARCH**

# Testing and Counseling: BRCA Mutations and Beyond

Genetic testing for BRCA mutations and other hereditary cancer predisposition genes has transformed the landscape of cancer prevention, early detection, and treatment decision-making. In this comprehensive overview, we will delve into the significance of genetic testing, the complexities of counseling, implications of BRCA mutations, and advancements in identifying genetic susceptibility beyond BRCA.

**ADVANCEMENTS IN BREAST CANCER RESEARCH**

1. Importance of Genetic Testing:

Genetic testing has become a cornerstone in oncology, offering invaluable insights into an individual's inherited risk of developing certain cancers. Key aspects of the importance of genetic testing include:

- Personalized Risk Assessment: Genetic testing allows for personalized risk assessment, enabling individuals and their healthcare providers to tailor screening, prevention, and treatment strategies based on their unique genetic makeup and cancer risk profile.
- Early Detection and Prevention: Knowledge of genetic mutations facilitates early detection through enhanced surveillance protocols and preventive measures such as risk-reducing surgeries, chemoprevention, and lifestyle modifications, ultimately leading to better outcomes.
- Family Planning: Genetic testing results may influence family planning decisions, including

reproductive choices, prenatal testing, and adoption considerations, as individuals may want to make informed decisions about their family's health and future generations.
- Treatment Decision-Making: In certain cases, genetic testing results may impact treatment decisions, particularly in the context of targeted therapies or participation in clinical trials for individuals with specific genetic alterations.

2. Genetic Counseling Considerations:

Genetic counseling is an integral part of the genetic testing process, providing individuals and families with comprehensive education, support, and guidance. Important considerations in genetic counseling include:

- Pre-Test Counseling: Genetic counselors offer pre-test counseling to discuss the purpose of genetic testing, the potential outcomes, the implications of test results, and the psychosocial impact of genetic testing on individuals and their families.

- Family History Assessment: A detailed family history assessment is conducted to identify patterns of hereditary cancer risk, assess the likelihood of an inherited predisposition, and guide the selection of appropriate genetic testing strategies.
- Informed Decision-Making: Genetic counselors empower individuals to make informed decisions about genetic testing by providing accurate information, addressing misconceptions, clarifying risks and benefits, and respecting autonomy and personal values.
- Post-Test Counseling: Genetic counselors provide post-test counseling to interpret genetic testing results, discuss implications for medical management, recommend personalized risk reduction strategies, and offer psychosocial support to help individuals cope with the emotional and psychological impact of genetic testing results.
- Ethical and Legal Considerations: Genetic counselors address ethical and legal issues related to genetic testing, including privacy, confidentiality, genetic discrimination, and

**ADVANCEMENTS IN BREAST CANCER RESEARCH**
the implications of testing for insurance coverage and employment.

3. Implications of BRCA Mutations:

BRCA1 and BRCA2 are tumor suppressor genes involved in DNA repair and maintenance of genomic stability. Inherited mutations in BRCA1 or BRCA2 are associated with an increased risk of breast, ovarian, prostate, pancreatic, and other cancers. Key implications of BRCA mutations include:

- Hereditary Breast and Ovarian Cancer Syndrome (HBOC): BRCA mutations are the most well-known contributors to HBOC syndrome, a hereditary cancer predisposition syndrome characterized by an increased risk of breast and ovarian cancers in affected families.
- Elevated Cancer Risk: Individuals with BRCA1 or BRCA2 mutations have a

significantly elevated risk of developing breast and ovarian cancers compared to the general population, with lifetime risks estimated to be up to 70-80% for breast cancer and 40-60% for ovarian cancer.
- Risk-Reducing Strategies: Knowledge of BRCA mutations allows for risk-reducing strategies such as enhanced surveillance (e.g., breast MRI, transvaginal ultrasound), risk-reducing surgeries (e.g., prophylactic mastectomy, salpingo-oophorectomy), and chemoprevention (e.g., tamoxifen, oral contraceptives) to reduce the risk of cancer development or detect cancer at an early, more treatable stage.
- Family Screening: Identification of BRCA mutations in an individual has implications for their family members, who may also be at increased risk of carrying the mutation and developing cancer. Family screening and genetic testing are recommended for at-risk relatives to identify carriers and implement appropriate risk management strategies.

4. Advancements Beyond BRCA:

**ADVANCEMENTS IN BREAST CANCER RESEARCH**

While BRCA mutations are well-established contributors to hereditary cancer risk, advancements in genetic testing technology have expanded our understanding of other cancer susceptibility genes and hereditary cancer syndromes. Key advancements beyond BRCA include:

- Multi-Gene Panel Testing: Multi-gene panel testing allows for simultaneous analysis of multiple cancer susceptibility genes, including genes associated with breast cancer (e.g., PALB2, CHEK2), ovarian cancer (e.g., BRIP1, RAD51C), Lynch syndrome, Li-Fraumeni syndrome, and other hereditary cancer syndromes. Multi-gene panel testing provides a more comprehensive assessment of inherited cancer risk and may identify mutations in genes beyond BRCA.
- Polygenic Risk Scores: Polygenic risk scores (PRS) incorporate information from multiple common genetic variants across the genome

## ADVANCEMENTS IN BREAST CANCER RESEARCH

to estimate an individual's overall genetic susceptibility to cancer. PRS may complement traditional genetic testing by identifying individuals at increased risk of cancer who do not carry pathogenic mutations in known cancer susceptibility.

**ADVANCEMENTS IN BREAST CANCER RESEARCH**

# Therapies in Breast Cancer: HER2-Targeted Agents, Hormonal Therapies, and PARP Inhibitors

Breast cancer is a complex disease with various subtypes characterized by distinct molecular profiles. Treatment strategies are tailored based on the molecular characteristics of the tumor, and targeted therapies have emerged as a cornerstone in breast cancer management. In this comprehensive overview, we will discuss three major classes of targeted therapies: HER2-targeted agents, hormonal therapies, and PARP inhibitors.

1. HER2-Targeted Agents:

**ADVANCEMENTS IN BREAST CANCER RESEARCH**

Human Epidermal Growth Factor Receptor 2 (HER2) is a cell surface receptor that plays a crucial role in cell growth, proliferation, and survival. Approximately 15-20% of breast cancers overexpress HER2, which is associated with aggressive tumor behavior and poorer prognosis. HER2-targeted agents specifically inhibit HER2 signaling pathways, leading to tumor growth inhibition and improved outcomes in HER2-positive breast cancer.

Key HER2-Targeted Agents:

- Trastuzumab (Herceptin): Trastuzumab was the first HER2-targeted monoclonal antibody approved for the treatment of HER2-positive breast cancer. It binds to the extracellular domain of the HER2 receptor, inhibiting downstream signaling pathways and inducing antibody-dependent cellular cytotoxicity (ADCC). Trastuzumab is used in both early and metastatic settings, often in combination with chemotherapy, and has significantly improved survival outcomes in HER2-positive breast cancer patients.
- Pertuzumab (Perjeta): Pertuzumab is another HER2-targeted monoclonal antibody

that inhibits HER2 signaling by binding to a different epitope on the HER2 receptor compared to trastuzumab. It prevents heterodimerization of HER2 with other HER family members, such as HER3, leading to more effective blockade of downstream signaling pathways. Pertuzumab is typically used in combination with trastuzumab and chemotherapy as neoadjuvant and metastatic treatment for HER2-positive breast cancer.

- Ado-Trastuzumab Emtansine (T-DM1): T-DM1 is an antibody-drug conjugate that combines trastuzumab with the cytotoxic agent emtansine (DM1). It delivers cytotoxic payload directly to HER2-positive cancer cells, resulting in targeted cell death. T-DM1 is indicated for the treatment of HER2-positive metastatic breast cancer that has progressed after prior trastuzumab-based therapy and has shown superior efficacy and tolerability compared to standard chemotherapy in this setting.
- Lapatinib: Lapatinib is a small molecule tyrosine kinase inhibitor (TKI) that inhibits both HER2 and epidermal growth factor receptor (EGFR) tyrosine kinases. It blocks HER2 and EGFR signaling pathways,

leading to cell cycle arrest and apoptosis. Lapatinib is used in combination with chemotherapy for the treatment of HER2-positive metastatic breast cancer, particularly in patients who have progressed on trastuzumab-based therapy.

2. Hormonal Therapies:

Hormone receptor-positive breast cancers express estrogen receptor (ER) and/or progesterone receptor (PR) and are dependent on estrogen signaling for growth and survival. Hormonal therapies target ER and/or PR signaling pathways, either by blocking estrogen production or by inhibiting estrogen receptor activity, thereby suppressing tumor growth and delaying disease progression in hormone receptor-positive breast cancer.

Key Hormonal Therapies:

- Selective Estrogen Receptor Modulators (SERMs): SERMs such as tamoxifen and raloxifene bind to the estrogen receptor and modulate its activity, acting as estrogen agonists or antagonists depending on the tissue type. Tamoxifen is a cornerstone of adjuvant hormonal therapy for premenopausal and postmenopausal women with hormone receptor-positive breast cancer and has been shown to reduce the risk of recurrence and improve survival outcomes.

- Aromatase Inhibitors (AIs): AIs block the conversion of androgens to estrogens by inhibiting the enzyme aromatase, which is responsible for estrogen synthesis in postmenopausal women. AIs include non-steroidal AIs (e.g., letrozole, anastrozole) and steroidal AIs (e.g., exemestane). AIs are used as adjuvant or metastatic treatment options for postmenopausal women with hormone receptor-positive breast cancer and have demonstrated superior efficacy compared to tamoxifen in certain settings.
- Selective Estrogen Receptor Degraders (SERDs): SERDs such as fulvestrant bind to the estrogen receptor and induce its degradation, leading to complete suppression of estrogen receptor signaling. Fulvestrant is indicated for the treatment of hormone receptor-positive metastatic breast

cancer in postmenopausal women who have progressed on prior endocrine therapy and has shown efficacy in delaying disease progression and improving survival outcomes.

3. PARP Inhibitors:

Poly (ADP-ribose) polymerase (PARP) inhibitors are a class of targeted therapies that exploit synthetic lethality in tumors with homologous recombination deficiency (HRD), including those with BRCA mutations. PARP inhibitors block the activity of PARP enzymes, which are involved in DNA repair mechanisms, leading to the accumulation of DNA damage and cell death in cancer cells with impaired DNA repair capacity.

Key PARP Inhibitors:

- Olaparib: Olaparib was the first PARP inhibitor approved for the treatment of metastatic breast cancer with BRCA mutations. It has shown efficacy in both germline and somatic BRCA-mutated breast cancers, significantly improving

**ADVANCEMENTS IN BREAST CANCER RESEARCH**

progression-free survival and overall survival compared to standard chemotherapy in this population.

- Talazoparib: Talazoparib is another PARP inhibitor approved for the treatment of metastatic breast cancer with germline BRCA mutations. It has demonstrated superior efficacy and tolerability compared to standard chemotherapy, with a significant improvement in progression-free survival and a higher overall response rate in BRCA-mutated breast cancers.

ADVANCEMENTS IN BREAST CANCER RESEARCH

# Mechanisms of Action, Resistance, and Novel Approaches in Breast Cancer Treatment

Breast cancer treatment has undergone significant advancements in recent years, with a deeper understanding of the disease's molecular mechanisms leading to the development of targeted therapies. Despite these advances, resistance to treatment remains a challenge, necessitating ongoing research into novel therapeutic approaches. In this comprehensive overview, we will delve into the mechanisms of action of existing therapies, explore mechanisms of resistance, and discuss emerging novel approaches in breast cancer treatment.

**ADVANCEMENTS IN BREAST CANCER RESEARCH**

1. Mechanisms of Action:

HER2-Targeted Agents: HER2-targeted therapies, such as trastuzumab and pertuzumab, work by inhibiting HER2 signaling pathways, leading to cell cycle arrest, apoptosis, and inhibition of tumor growth. Trastuzumab exerts its effects through antibody-dependent cellular cytotoxicity (ADCC), while pertuzumab prevents HER2 heterodimerization with other HER family members.

Hormonal Therapies: Hormonal therapies, including selective estrogen receptor modulators (SERMs) like tamoxifen and aromatase inhibitors (AIs) like letrozole, work by blocking estrogen signaling in hormone receptor-positive breast cancer. Tamoxifen competes with estrogen for binding to the estrogen receptor, while AIs inhibit the production of estrogen by blocking aromatase enzyme activity.

PARP Inhibitors: PARP inhibitors, such as olaparib and talazoparib, exploit synthetic lethality in breast cancer cells with homologous recombination deficiency (HRD), including those with BRCA mutations. PARP inhibitors block the activity of PARP enzymes involved in DNA repair, leading to

**ADVANCEMENTS IN BREAST CANCER RESEARCH**

the accumulation of DNA damage and cell death in BRCA-mutated cancer cells.

2. Mechanisms of Resistance:

Despite the initial efficacy of targeted therapies, resistance often develops, limiting their long-term effectiveness. Mechanisms of resistance to breast cancer therapies include:

- HER2 Pathway Activation: Resistance to HER2-targeted therapies can occur through upregulation of alternative signaling pathways, such as the PI3K/AKT/mTOR pathway, leading to HER2-independent tumor growth.
- Estrogen Receptor Alterations: Resistance to hormonal therapies can arise from alterations in the estrogen receptor (ER) pathway, such as mutations in the ER gene or upregulation of alternative signaling pathways, resulting in estrogen-independent tumor growth.
- BRCA Reversion Mutations: Resistance to PARP inhibitors in BRCA-mutated breast cancers can occur through the acquisition of secondary mutations that restore

homologous recombination function, allowing cancer cells to repair DNA damage and survive PARP inhibition.
- Tumor Microenvironment Changes: The tumor microenvironment, including stromal cells, immune cells, and extracellular matrix components, can promote treatment resistance by providing survival signals to cancer cells, inducing immunosuppression, and facilitating metastasis.

3. Novel Approaches:

To overcome resistance and improve treatment outcomes in breast cancer, researchers are exploring several novel approaches, including:

- Combination Therapies: Combining targeted therapies with different mechanisms of action or with conventional chemotherapy agents can overcome resistance mechanisms and enhance treatment efficacy. For example, dual HER2 blockade with trastuzumab and pertuzumab has demonstrated improved outcomes compared to single-agent therapy in HER2-positive breast cancer.

- Immunotherapy: Immunotherapy, particularly immune checkpoint inhibitors targeting programmed death-ligand 1 (PD-L1) or cytotoxic T-lymphocyte-associated protein 4 (CTLA-4), has shown promising results in subsets of breast cancer patients, particularly those with triple-negative breast cancer (TNBC) or PD-L1-positive tumors.
- Precision Medicine: Advances in genomic profiling and molecular characterization of breast cancer tumors allow for more precise identification of molecular alterations driving tumor growth and progression. Precision medicine approaches enable personalized treatment strategies based on the unique molecular profile of each patient's tumor.
- Targeting Tumor Microenvironment: Therapies targeting components of the tumor microenvironment, such as stromal cells, immune cells, and angiogenic factors, hold promise for disrupting tumor-promoting signals and enhancing the anti-tumor immune response.
- Therapeutic Vaccines: Therapeutic cancer vaccines designed to stimulate the immune system to recognize and target

**ADVANCEMENTS IN BREAST CANCER RESEARCH**
tumor-specific antigens are being investigated as potential treatments for breast cancer, either as standalone therapies or in combination with other treatment modalities.

**ADVANCEMENTS IN BREAST CANCER RESEARCH**

# Radiation Therapy: Techniques, Fractionation Schedules, and Side Effects

Radiation therapy plays a crucial role in the treatment of breast cancer, serving as an effective adjuvant therapy following surgery to eradicate residual tumor cells and reduce the risk of local recurrence. In this comprehensive overview, we will discuss various techniques of radiation therapy, fractionation schedules commonly used in breast cancer treatment, and potential side effects associated with this modality.

1. Techniques of Radiation Therapy:

    a. External Beam Radiation Therapy (EBRT):

**ADVANCEMENTS IN BREAST CANCER RESEARCH**

EBRT is the most common form of radiation therapy used in breast cancer treatment. It involves delivering high-energy radiation beams from an external machine to target the breast or chest wall. EBRT techniques include:

- 3D Conformal Radiation Therapy (3DCRT): 3DCRT uses multiple radiation beams aimed at the tumor from different angles, with customized blocking to spare surrounding healthy tissues. This technique ensures precise targeting of the tumor while minimizing radiation exposure to nearby organs.
- Intensity-Modulated Radiation Therapy (IMRT): IMRT delivers radiation with varying intensities across the treatment field, allowing for more precise dose modulation and sparing of critical structures. IMRT is particularly useful for treating complex tumor shapes or cases where organs at risk are close to the target area.
- Volumetric Modulated Arc Therapy (VMAT): VMAT is a type of IMRT that delivers radiation in a continuous arc around the patient, enabling highly conformal dose

distributions with shorter treatment times compared to traditional IMRT techniques.

b. Intraoperative Radiation Therapy (IORT):

IORT involves delivering a single high dose of radiation directly to the tumor bed during surgery, immediately following tumor resection. This technique offers the advantage of delivering radiation to the target area while sparing surrounding healthy tissues, reducing treatment duration, and minimizing side effects.

c. Brachytherapy:

Brachytherapy involves the placement of radioactive sources directly within or near the tumor site. In breast cancer treatment, brachytherapy can be delivered as either:

- Interstitial Brachytherapy: Radioactive seeds or catheters are implanted directly into the breast tissue surrounding the tumor bed, delivering localized radiation therapy over a specified treatment period.

- Intracavitary Brachytherapy: A balloon catheter is placed within the surgical cavity of the breast, and a radioactive source is temporarily inserted into the balloon to deliver radiation to the surrounding tissues.

2. Fractionation Schedules:

Fractionation refers to the division of the total radiation dose into smaller doses, delivered over multiple treatment sessions (fractions), to maximize tumor control while minimizing damage to healthy tissues. Common fractionation schedules used in breast cancer treatment include:

- Conventional Fractionation: In conventional fractionation, patients typically receive daily radiation treatments (Monday to Friday) over a period of 5 to 7 weeks, with each treatment session lasting a few minutes. The total radiation dose is divided into smaller fractions (usually 1.8 to 2 Gy per fraction) to allow for normal tissue repair between treatments.

**ADVANCEMENTS IN BREAST CANCER RESEARCH**

- Hypofractionation: Hypofractionation involves delivering higher doses of radiation per fraction over a shorter treatment duration, typically 3 to 4 weeks. This approach aims to reduce overall treatment time and healthcare costs while maintaining equivalent tumor control rates and cosmetic outcomes. Hypofractionated regimens commonly used in breast cancer treatment include 40 Gy in 15 fractions or 42.5 Gy in 16 fractions.
- Accelerated Partial Breast Irradiation (APBI): APBI delivers radiation specifically to the tumor bed or lumpectomy cavity, sparing the surrounding breast tissue. This approach allows for a shorter treatment course (typically 5 to 10 days) with higher doses per fraction, minimizing radiation exposure to healthy tissues and reducing treatment-related toxicity.

3. Side Effects of Radiation Therapy:

While radiation therapy is highly effective in controlling tumor growth and reducing the risk of local recurrence, it can also cause side effects due to radiation exposure of normal tissues surrounding

**ADVANCEMENTS IN BREAST CANCER RESEARCH**
the treatment area. Common side effects of radiation therapy for breast cancer include:

- Skin Irritation: Radiation therapy can cause redness, itching, and irritation of the skin in the treated area, resembling a sunburn. Skin reactions typically occur within a few weeks of starting treatment and may worsen over the course of therapy before gradually improving after treatment completion.
- Fatigue: Radiation therapy can cause fatigue, which may persist throughout the treatment course and for several weeks to months afterward. Fatigue can affect daily activities and quality of life and may require adjustments to daily routines and activities.
- Breast Changes: Radiation therapy can lead to changes in breast appearance and texture, including swelling, firmness, and fibrosis (thickening and hardening of breast tissue). These changes may be temporary or permanent and can affect breast symmetry and cosmesis.
- Lymphedema: Radiation therapy to the axillary lymph nodes can increase the risk of lymphedema, a condition characterized by swelling and fluid accumulation in the arm or

chest wall. Lymphedema may occur months to years after radiation treatment and can be managed with compression garments, physical therapy, and lifestyle modifications.
- Cardiac Toxicity: Radiation therapy to the left breast or chest wall may pose a risk of cardiac toxicity, particularly in patients with pre-existing cardiovascular risk factors. Long-term follow-up studies have shown an increased risk of cardiac events, such as myocardial infarction and cardiomyopathy, following radiation therapy to the left breast.
- Pulmonary Toxicity: Radiation therapy to the chest wall or internal mammary lymph nodes may increase the risk of pulmonary toxicity, including radiation pneumonitis and fibrosis. Symptoms may include cough, shortness of breath, and chest pain, and can occur months to years after radiation treatment.

ADVANCEMENTS IN BREAST CANCER RESEARCH

# Immunotherapy in Breast Cancer: Checkpoint Inhibitors, CAR-T Cells, and Vaccines

Immunotherapy has emerged as a promising treatment modality in breast cancer, offering a novel approach to harness the body's immune system to target and eliminate cancer cells. In this comprehensive overview, we will discuss the various immunotherapy strategies employed in breast cancer treatment, including checkpoint inhibitors, chimeric antigen receptor (CAR) T-cell therapy, and therapeutic vaccines.

1. Checkpoint Inhibitors:

Checkpoint inhibitors are monoclonal antibodies that target immune checkpoint proteins, such as programmed death-ligand 1 (PD-L1) and cytotoxic T-lymphocyte-associated protein 4 (CTLA-4), which

## ADVANCEMENTS IN BREAST CANCER RESEARCH

regulate the activity of T cells in the immune system. By blocking these checkpoints, checkpoint inhibitors enhance the ability of T cells to recognize and destroy cancer cells.

Key Checkpoint Inhibitors in Breast Cancer:

- Pembrolizumab: Pembrolizumab is a PD-1 inhibitor approved for the treatment of metastatic triple-negative breast cancer (TNBC) that expresses PD-L1. Clinical trials have shown promising results with pembrolizumab in combination with chemotherapy as first-line treatment for PD-L1-positive metastatic TNBC, leading to improved progression-free survival and overall survival compared to chemotherapy alone.
- Atezolizumab: Atezolizumab is a PD-L1 inhibitor approved for use in combination with nab-paclitaxel chemotherapy for the treatment of unresectable locally advanced or metastatic TNBC that expresses PD-L1. Clinical trials have demonstrated improved progression-free survival and overall survival with atezolizumab plus nab-paclitaxel

compared to chemotherapy alone in PD-L1-positive TNBC.
- Durvalumab: Durvalumab is another PD-L1 inhibitor being evaluated in clinical trials for the treatment of breast cancer, both as monotherapy and in combination with other agents. Preliminary data suggest potential efficacy in certain subsets of breast cancer patients, particularly those with TNBC.

2. CAR-T Cell Therapy:

CAR-T cell therapy is a form of adoptive cell therapy that involves genetically modifying a patient's T cells to express chimeric antigen receptors (CARs) targeting specific tumor antigens. Once infused back into the patient, CAR-T cells recognize and eliminate cancer cells expressing the target antigen.

CAR-T Cell Therapy Targets in Breast Cancer:

- HER2: HER2-targeted CAR-T cell therapy has shown promise in preclinical studies and early-phase clinical trials for HER2-positive breast cancer. By targeting

HER2-expressing tumor cells, CAR-T cells can induce tumor regression and improve survival outcomes in patients with advanced HER2-positive breast cancer.

3. Therapeutic Vaccines:

Therapeutic cancer vaccines are designed to stimulate the immune system to recognize and attack tumor-specific antigens, leading to targeted destruction of cancer cells. Vaccines can be based on tumor-associated antigens (TAAs) or tumor-specific antigens (TSAs) expressed exclusively by cancer cells.

Types of Therapeutic Vaccines in Breast Cancer:

- HER2 Vaccines: HER2-targeted therapeutic vaccines aim to induce an immune response against HER2-expressing breast cancer cells. Vaccines may contain HER2 peptides, proteins, or DNA fragments, combined with adjuvants to enhance immune activation.
- MUC1 Vaccines: Mucin 1 (MUC1) is a glycoprotein overexpressed in many breast cancers, making it an attractive target for

therapeutic vaccination. MUC1-based vaccines aim to elicit immune responses against MUC1-expressing tumor cells, leading to tumor regression and improved outcomes.
- Neoantigen Vaccines: Neoantigens are tumor-specific antigens derived from somatic mutations in cancer cells. Neoantigen-based vaccines are personalized therapies that target patient-specific mutations, enhancing immune recognition of tumor cells and inducing tumor-specific immune responses.

Clinical Challenges and Future Directions:

While immunotherapy has shown promising results in certain subsets of breast cancer patients, challenges remain, including:

- Biomarker Identification: Identifying reliable predictive biomarkers of response to immunotherapy remains a challenge in breast cancer. Biomarkers such as PD-L1 expression and tumor mutational burden (TMB) have shown some utility but may not capture the full spectrum of responders.

**ADVANCEMENTS IN BREAST CANCER RESEARCH**

- Combination Therapies: Combining immunotherapy with other treatment modalities, such as chemotherapy, targeted therapy, or radiation therapy, may enhance treatment efficacy and overcome resistance mechanisms. Rational combinations based on preclinical and clinical data are under investigation.
- Patient Selection: Identifying patients most likely to benefit from immunotherapy remains a key clinical challenge. Patient selection based on tumor molecular subtype, immune infiltrate profile, and other biomarkers of response is critical for optimizing treatment outcomes.
- Overcoming Resistance: Resistance to immunotherapy can develop through various mechanisms, including upregulation of alternative immune checkpoints, tumor immune evasion mechanisms, and immunosuppressive tumor microenvironment. Strategies to overcome resistance are being investigated, including combination therapies and immune modulatory agents.

# Precision Medicine in Breast Cancer Treatment: Molecular Profiling and Personalized Therapies

Precision medicine in breast cancer treatment represents a paradigm shift towards tailoring therapeutic approaches based on the unique molecular characteristics of each patient's tumor. Molecular profiling techniques allow clinicians to identify specific genetic alterations, gene expression patterns, and molecular subtypes that drive tumor growth and progression. This comprehensive overview will explore the principles of precision medicine in breast cancer treatment, including molecular profiling technologies, molecular subtyping, and personalized therapeutic strategies.

1. Molecular Profiling Technologies:

## ADVANCEMENTS IN BREAST CANCER RESEARCH

a. Next-Generation Sequencing (NGS): NGS enables comprehensive genomic analysis of breast cancer tumors, allowing for the identification of somatic mutations, copy number alterations, and gene expression patterns. Whole-genome sequencing (WGS), whole-exome sequencing (WES), and targeted sequencing panels are commonly used NGS approaches in molecular profiling.

b. Gene Expression Profiling: Gene expression profiling techniques, such as microarray-based assays and RNA sequencing, measure the expression levels of thousands of genes in breast cancer tumors. These assays provide insights into the molecular subtypes of breast cancer and can help predict prognosis and treatment response.

c. DNA Methylation Profiling: DNA methylation profiling assesses changes in DNA methylation patterns associated with breast cancer development and progression. Methylation arrays and bisulfite sequencing are commonly used techniques to identify aberrant DNA methylation patterns in breast cancer tumors.

d. Proteomic and Metabolomic Profiling: Proteomic and metabolomic profiling techniques analyze

**ADVANCEMENTS IN BREAST CANCER RESEARCH**
protein and metabolite expression patterns in breast cancer tumors, providing insights into dysregulated signaling pathways and metabolic alterations associated with tumor growth and progression.

2. Molecular Subtyping of Breast Cancer:

a. Luminal Subtypes: Luminal breast cancers are characterized by the expression of hormone receptors (estrogen receptor [ER] and/or progesterone receptor [PR]) and low expression of HER2. Luminal A tumors typically have low proliferation rates and better prognosis, while luminal B tumors are more proliferative and associated with poorer outcomes.

b. HER2-Enriched Subtype: HER2-enriched breast cancers overexpress the HER2 receptor and are associated with aggressive tumor behavior. HER2-targeted therapies, such as trastuzumab and pertuzumab, are effective treatments for HER2-positive breast cancer.

c. Basal-like/Triple-Negative Subtype: Basal-like or triple-negative breast cancers lack expression of hormone receptors (ER, PR) and HER2 amplification. These tumors are associated with high proliferation rates, early recurrence, and poor prognosis. Chemotherapy remains the mainstay of treatment for triple-negative breast cancer.

d. Claudin-Low Subtype: Claudin-low breast cancers are characterized by low expression of cell-cell adhesion molecules (claudins) and immune cell infiltration. These tumors are associated with mesenchymal features, stem cell-like properties, and resistance to chemotherapy.

3. Personalized Therapeutic Strategies:

a. Hormonal Therapies: Hormonal therapies, such as selective estrogen receptor modulators (SERMs), aromatase inhibitors (AIs), and selective estrogen receptor downregulators (SERDs), target the estrogen receptor signaling pathway in hormone receptor-positive breast cancer. Molecular profiling helps identify patients who are most likely to benefit from hormonal therapies based on their tumor's hormone receptor status and gene expression profile.

b. HER2-Targeted Therapies: HER2-targeted therapies, including monoclonal antibodies (trastuzumab, pertuzumab), antibody-drug conjugates (T-DM1), and small molecule tyrosine

**ADVANCEMENTS IN BREAST CANCER RESEARCH**

kinase inhibitors (lapatinib), are effective treatments for HER2-positive breast cancer. Molecular profiling helps identify patients with HER2 overexpression or amplification who are candidates for HER2-targeted therapy.

c. PARP Inhibitors: PARP inhibitors, such as olaparib and talazoparib, target DNA repair pathways in breast cancers with homologous recombination deficiency (HRD), including those with BRCA mutations. Molecular profiling helps identify patients with HRD tumors who are likely to benefit from PARP inhibitor therapy.

d. Immunotherapy: Immunotherapy approaches, such as immune checkpoint inhibitors (e.g., pembrolizumab) and CAR-T cell therapy, harness the immune system to target and eliminate cancer cells. Molecular profiling helps identify patients with immune-infiltrated tumors or high tumor mutational burden (TMB) who are candidates for immunotherapy.

4. Challenges and Future Directions:

a. Tumor Heterogeneity: Intra-tumoral and inter-tumoral heterogeneity pose challenges for molecular profiling and personalized treatment

# ADVANCEMENTS IN BREAST CANCER RESEARCH

strategies. Single-site biopsies may not capture the full spectrum of genetic alterations and molecular subtypes present within a patient's tumor, necessitating the development of techniques to assess tumor heterogeneity comprehensively.

b. Resistance Mechanisms: Acquired resistance to targeted therapies and immunotherapies remains a significant clinical challenge in breast cancer treatment. Understanding the molecular mechanisms underlying resistance and developing strategies to overcome resistance are critical for improving treatment outcomes and long-term survival.

c. Integration of Multi-Omics Data: Integrating data from multiple omics platforms (genomics, transcriptomics, proteomics, metabolomics) holds promise for a more comprehensive understanding of breast cancer biology and the identification of novel therapeutic targets. Advances in computational biology and bioinformatics are facilitating the integration and analysis of multi-omics data to guide personalized treatment approaches.

d. Clinical Implementation: Translating molecular profiling findings into clinical practice requires

**ADVANCEMENTS IN BREAST CANCER RESEARCH**
standardized assays, robust biomarkers, and evidence-based guidelines for treatment selection. Clinical trials are essential for validating the clinical utility of molecular profiling assays and establishing their role in guiding personalized treatment decisions.

ADVANCEMENTS IN BREAST CANCER RESEARCH

# Clinical Trials in Breast Cancer: Design, Implementation, and Ethical Considerations

Clinical trials play a pivotal role in advancing the field of breast cancer treatment by evaluating the safety and efficacy of new therapeutic approaches, improving patient outcomes, and guiding evidence-based clinical practice. In this comprehensive overview, we will explore the design, implementation, and ethical considerations of clinical trials in breast cancer research.

1. Design of Clinical Trials:

a. Study Objectives: Clinical trials in breast cancer may aim to assess various endpoints, including overall survival, progression-free survival, response rates, quality of life, and safety profiles of investigational treatments. Study objectives are

**ADVANCEMENTS IN BREAST CANCER RESEARCH**
defined based on the research question and the specific goals of the trial.

b. Study Design: Clinical trials can be categorized into several design types, including:

- Randomized Controlled Trials (RCTs): RCTs compare the outcomes of patients receiving the investigational treatment(s) with those receiving standard-of-care treatment or placebo. Randomization helps minimize bias and ensure the comparability of treatment groups.
- Phase I Trials: Phase I trials evaluate the safety, tolerability, and dose escalation of investigational drugs in a small cohort of patients to determine the maximum tolerated dose (MTD) and recommended phase II dose (RP2D).
- Phase II Trials: Phase II trials assess the preliminary efficacy of investigational treatments in larger patient cohorts, typically focusing on specific tumor types or molecular subgroups.
- Phase III Trials: Phase III trials compare the efficacy and safety of investigational treatments with standard-of-care treatments

# ADVANCEMENTS IN BREAST CANCER RESEARCH

in large patient populations to establish clinical benefit and support regulatory approval.

c. Endpoints and Outcome Measures: Clinical trials in breast cancer may utilize various endpoints to evaluate treatment efficacy and safety, including:

- Primary Endpoints: Primary endpoints measure the main outcome of interest, such as overall survival, progression-free survival, or objective response rate.
- Secondary Endpoints: Secondary endpoints assess additional treatment outcomes, such as quality of life, duration of response, time to progression, and biomarker analyses.
- Exploratory Endpoints: Exploratory endpoints explore novel aspects of treatment response or mechanism of action, such as pharmacokinetics, pharmacodynamics, and correlative biomarker studies.

d. Statistical Considerations: Sample size calculation, randomization procedures, and statistical analysis plans are critical components of

**ADVANCEMENTS IN BREAST CANCER RESEARCH**

clinical trial design. Power calculations ensure that the study has sufficient statistical power to detect clinically meaningful differences between treatment groups, while randomization minimizes selection bias and confounding factors.

2. Implementation of Clinical Trials:

a. Patient Recruitment and Informed Consent: Patient recruitment is essential for the successful conduct of clinical trials. Recruitment strategies may involve collaboration with multiple healthcare institutions, patient advocacy groups, and community outreach programs. Informed consent is obtained from all study participants, outlining the trial objectives, procedures, risks, benefits, and voluntary nature of participation.

b. Treatment Administration and Monitoring: Investigational treatments are administered according to the study protocol, with careful monitoring of treatment adherence, adverse events, and treatment response. Clinical trial protocols include guidelines for patient evaluation, treatment dosing, toxicity management, and follow-up assessments.

c. Data Collection and Management: Clinical trial data are collected using standardized case report forms (CRFs) and electronic data capture (EDC) systems. Data management procedures ensure the accuracy, completeness, and confidentiality of patient information throughout the trial. Quality control measures, such as source data verification and monitoring visits, are implemented to maintain data integrity.

d. Safety Monitoring and Reporting: Safety monitoring is a critical aspect of clinical trial conduct, involving ongoing assessment of treatment-related adverse events and serious adverse events (SAEs). Adverse events are graded according to standardized criteria (e.g., Common Terminology Criteria for Adverse Events [CTCAE]), and SAEs are promptly reported to regulatory authorities, institutional review boards (IRBs), and data safety monitoring boards (DSMBs).

3. Ethical Considerations:

a. Institutional Review Board (IRB) Approval: Clinical trials must receive ethical approval from an IRB or ethics committee before initiation. IRBs review study protocols to ensure patient safety, scientific validity, and compliance with ethical

## ADVANCEMENTS IN BREAST CANCER RESEARCH

principles, including respect for patient autonomy, beneficence, non-maleficence, and justice.

b. Informed Consent: Informed consent is a fundamental ethical principle in clinical research, requiring that patients are adequately informed about the purpose, risks, benefits, and alternatives of participation in a clinical trial. Informed consent documents should be written in a clear, understandable language and obtained voluntarily without coercion.

c. Benefit-Risk Assessment: Clinical trials should balance the potential benefits of investigational treatments with the risks to patient safety and well-being. Benefit-risk assessments consider factors such as the severity of the disease, availability of alternative treatments, potential toxicity of investigational agents, and likelihood of therapeutic benefit.

d. Data Integrity and Transparency: Maintaining data integrity and transparency is essential for ensuring the reliability and credibility of clinical trial results. Clinical trial sponsors, investigators, and regulatory agencies are responsible for accurately reporting study findings, disclosing conflicts of interest, and adhering to data-sharing policies.

**ADVANCEMENTS IN BREAST CANCER RESEARCH**

4. Challenges and Future Directions:

a. Patient Access and Participation: Access to clinical trials remains a challenge for many patients, particularly those from underrepresented populations, rural areas, or low-income communities. Efforts to improve patient access and participation in clinical trials include expanding clinical trial eligibility criteria, reducing logistical barriers, and increasing patient education and awareness.

b. Biomarker-Driven Trials: Biomarker-driven clinical trials utilize molecular profiling data to identify patient subpopulations most likely to benefit from targeted therapies. Biomarker-guided treatment strategies improve treatment efficacy, minimize unnecessary toxicity, and optimize patient outcomes.

c. Adaptive Trial Designs: Adaptive trial designs allow for real-time modifications to study protocols based on accumulating data, enabling more efficient and flexible trial conduct. Adaptive designs can enhance patient enrollment, optimize treatment regimens, and accelerate the pace of clinical research.

**ADVANCEMENTS IN BREAST CANCER RESEARCH**

d. Collaborative Research Networks: Collaborative research networks, such as academic consortia, cooperative groups, and international alliances, facilitate multi-center clinical trials, data sharing, and collaborative research efforts. Collaborative networks promote scientific collaboration, accelerate knowledge dissemination, and foster innovation in breast cancer research.

ADVANCEMENTS IN BREAST CANCER RESEARCH

# Supportive Care and Survivorship: Managing Treatment Side Effects and Quality of Life Issues

Supportive care and survivorship play crucial roles in breast cancer treatment, focusing on managing treatment side effects and addressing quality of life issues to optimize patient outcomes. This comprehensive overview will explore various aspects of supportive care and survivorship in breast cancer, including the management of treatment-related side effects, psychosocial support, rehabilitation services, and survivorship care planning.

1. Managing Treatment Side Effects:

## ADVANCEMENTS IN BREAST CANCER RESEARCH

a. Chemotherapy-Related Side Effects:

- Nausea and Vomiting: Antiemetic medications, such as 5-HT3 receptor antagonists and NK1 receptor antagonists, can help prevent and alleviate chemotherapy-induced nausea and vomiting.
- Fatigue: Fatigue is a common side effect of chemotherapy. Energy conservation strategies, physical activity, and psychosocial support can help manage fatigue and improve energy levels.
- Peripheral Neuropathy: Neuropathic pain and tingling sensations in the hands and feet (peripheral neuropathy) may occur as a side effect of certain chemotherapy drugs. Symptomatic management with pain medications and physical therapy may be necessary.

b. Radiation Therapy-Related Side Effects:

- Skin Irritation: Radiation dermatitis, characterized by redness, itching, and skin irritation, is a common side effect of radiation

therapy. Topical emollients, corticosteroids, and dressings can help alleviate skin symptoms.
- Fatigue: Radiation therapy can cause fatigue, similar to chemotherapy-induced fatigue. Patients should be encouraged to rest when needed and engage in light physical activity to combat fatigue.

c. Hormonal Therapy-Related Side Effects:

- Hot Flashes: Hormonal therapies, such as tamoxifen and aromatase inhibitors, can induce hot flashes and night sweats. Lifestyle modifications, relaxation techniques, and pharmacological interventions (e.g., selective serotonin reuptake inhibitors [SSRIs]) can help manage vasomotor symptoms.
- Bone Health: Hormonal therapies may increase the risk of osteoporosis and bone fractures. Calcium and vitamin D supplementation, weight-bearing exercises, and bisphosphonate or denosumab therapy may be recommended to maintain bone health.

**ADVANCEMENTS IN BREAST CANCER RESEARCH**

2. Psychosocial Support:

a. Counseling and Psychotherapy: Psychosocial support services, including individual counseling, group therapy, and cognitive-behavioral therapy, can help patients cope with emotional distress, anxiety, depression, and adjustment to cancer diagnosis and treatment.

b. Support Groups: Peer support groups provide opportunities for patients to connect with others who have similar experiences, share coping strategies, and receive emotional support from fellow survivors.

c. Mind-Body Interventions: Mind-body interventions, such as mindfulness-based stress reduction (MBSR), yoga, meditation, and relaxation techniques, promote relaxation, stress reduction, and emotional well-being.

d. Social Work Services: Social workers play a vital role in addressing practical and financial concerns, accessing community resources, and providing assistance with transportation, housing, and insurance navigation.

3. Rehabilitation Services:

## ADVANCEMENTS IN BREAST CANCER RESEARCH

a. Physical Therapy: Physical therapists can help breast cancer survivors manage functional impairments, range of motion deficits, lymphedema, and musculoskeletal pain through tailored exercise programs, manual therapy techniques, and lymphedema management strategies.

b. Occupational Therapy: Occupational therapists assist patients in regaining independence in daily activities, such as self-care, work, and leisure pursuits, following breast cancer treatment. Adaptive equipment, ergonomic modifications, and energy conservation techniques may be recommended.

c. Speech Therapy: Speech-language pathologists provide evaluation and treatment for speech, swallowing, and vocal function issues that may arise as a result of breast cancer treatment, particularly in cases involving surgery or radiation therapy to the head and neck region.

4. Survivorship Care Planning:

a. Comprehensive Survivorship Care: Survivorship care planning involves addressing the ongoing physical, psychosocial, and supportive care needs of breast cancer survivors beyond the completion of

**ADVANCEMENTS IN BREAST CANCER RESEARCH**
active treatment. Survivorship care plans outline follow-up care guidelines, surveillance schedules, and recommendations for health maintenance and lifestyle interventions.

b. Late Effects Monitoring: Breast cancer survivors may experience long-term and late effects of treatment, such as cardiovascular complications, cognitive impairment, fertility issues, and secondary malignancies. Regular monitoring, screening, and early intervention are essential for detecting and managing late effects effectively.

c. Health Promotion and Wellness: Survivorship care emphasizes health promotion and wellness interventions, including smoking cessation, weight management, physical activity promotion, healthy diet counseling, and cancer screening recommendations (e.g., mammography, bone densitometry).

d. Coordination of Care: Survivorship care planning involves coordination and communication among primary care providers, oncology specialists, rehabilitation professionals, and support services to ensure comprehensive, patient-centered care.

ADVANCEMENTS IN BREAST CANCER RESEARCH

# Integrative Approaches to Breast Cancer Management: Nutrition, Exercise, and Mind-Body Therapies

Integrative approaches to breast cancer management involve combining conventional medical treatments with complementary and alternative therapies to address the physical, emotional, and psychosocial aspects of the disease. These approaches aim to optimize patient outcomes, enhance quality of life, and support overall well-being throughout the cancer journey. In this extensive overview, we will delve into the role of nutrition, exercise, and mind-body therapies in integrative breast cancer management.

1. Nutrition:

**ADVANCEMENTS IN BREAST CANCER RESEARCH**

a. Dietary Considerations:

- Balanced Diet: A balanced diet rich in fruits, vegetables, whole grains, lean proteins, and healthy fats is essential for overall health and well-being. Nutrient-dense foods provide essential vitamins, minerals, antioxidants, and phytochemicals that support immune function, reduce inflammation, and promote healing.
- Hydration: Staying hydrated is important for managing treatment side effects, such as nausea, fatigue, and dehydration. Patients should aim to drink plenty of fluids, including water, herbal teas, and electrolyte-rich beverages.
- Individualized Approach: Nutritional needs may vary among breast cancer patients based on treatment regimens, side effects, metabolic status, and personal preferences. Individualized nutrition counseling with a registered dietitian can help patients develop tailored dietary plans to meet their specific needs and goals.

b. Managing Treatment Side Effects:

**ADVANCEMENTS IN BREAST CANCER RESEARCH**

- Nausea and Vomiting: Certain foods and beverages, such as ginger, peppermint, and herbal teas, may help alleviate nausea and vomiting associated with chemotherapy or radiation therapy. Eating small, frequent meals and avoiding strong odors or greasy foods can also be helpful.
- Weight Management: Some breast cancer treatments, such as hormonal therapies, may lead to weight gain or changes in body composition. Maintaining a healthy weight through portion control, mindful eating, and regular physical activity can support overall health and reduce the risk of treatment-related complications.
- Bone Health: Adequate intake of calcium and vitamin D is important for maintaining bone health and reducing the risk of osteoporosis, especially for patients receiving hormonal therapies. Calcium-rich foods, such as dairy products, leafy greens, and fortified foods, should be included in the diet, along with vitamin D supplements as needed.

c. Nutritional Supplements:

**ADVANCEMENTS IN BREAST CANCER RESEARCH**

- Antioxidants: Some studies suggest that antioxidants, such as vitamin C, vitamin E, and selenium, may have protective effects against cancer development and treatment-related side effects. However, the use of antioxidant supplements during cancer treatment remains controversial, as high doses may interfere with treatment efficacy or increase the risk of adverse effects. Patients should consult with their healthcare providers before starting any supplements.
- Omega-3 Fatty Acids: Omega-3 fatty acids found in fish oil and flaxseed oil have anti-inflammatory properties and may help reduce inflammation, improve immune function, and support cardiovascular health. Incorporating omega-3-rich foods or supplements into the diet may be beneficial for breast cancer patients, but individual needs and considerations should be taken into account.

2. Exercise:

a. Benefits of Exercise:

**ADVANCEMENTS IN BREAST CANCER RESEARCH**

- Physical Well-Being: Regular exercise helps improve cardiovascular fitness, muscle strength, flexibility, and overall physical function. It can also help reduce the risk of treatment-related side effects, such as fatigue, lymphedema, and joint pain.
- Emotional Well-Being: Exercise has positive effects on mental health and emotional well-being, reducing symptoms of anxiety, depression, and stress commonly experienced by breast cancer patients. Physical activity releases endorphins, neurotransmitters that promote feelings of happiness and well-being.
- Quality of Life: Engaging in regular physical activity can enhance quality of life and improve self-esteem, body image, and social connectedness, fostering a sense of empowerment and control over one's health.

b. Types of Exercise:

- Aerobic Exercise: Activities such as walking, jogging, cycling, swimming, and dancing increase heart rate and oxygen

consumption, improving cardiovascular fitness and endurance.
- Strength Training: Resistance exercises using body weight, free weights, resistance bands, or weight machines help build muscle strength, bone density, and functional capacity.
- Flexibility and Balance: Stretching, yoga, tai chi, and Pilates enhance flexibility, balance, and coordination, reducing the risk of falls and injuries and promoting overall mobility and well-being.

c. Exercise Guidelines:

- Individualized Approach: Exercise recommendations should be tailored to the individual's fitness level, treatment status, physical limitations, and personal preferences. Patients should start slowly and gradually increase the intensity, duration, and frequency of exercise sessions, listening to their bodies and adjusting their activity level as needed.
- Safety Precautions: Breast cancer patients should consult with their healthcare

providers before starting or modifying an exercise program, especially during active treatment. Exercise safety considerations may include avoiding high-impact activities, protecting against lymphedema, and monitoring for signs of overexertion or injury.

3. Mind-Body Therapies:

a. Stress Reduction and Relaxation Techniques:

- Mindfulness Meditation: Mindfulness-based practices cultivate present-moment awareness and nonjudgmental acceptance of thoughts, emotions, and sensations, reducing stress and promoting emotional resilience.
- Yoga: Yoga combines physical postures, breathwork, and meditation techniques to improve flexibility, strength, and relaxation, enhancing overall well-being and quality of life.
- Deep Breathing Exercises: Deep breathing exercises, such as diaphragmatic breathing and paced breathing, promote relaxation,

reduce anxiety, and improve oxygenation, supporting overall health and vitality.

b. Cognitive-Behavioral Interventions:

- Cognitive Restructuring: Cognitive-behavioral therapy (CBT) techniques help patients identify and challenge negative thought patterns, beliefs, and behaviors associated with stress, anxiety, and depression. By reframing negative thoughts and focusing on adaptive coping strategies, patients can improve their emotional well-being and resilience.
- Stress Management: Stress management techniques, such as progressive muscle relaxation, guided imagery, and biofeedback, teach patients how to cope with stress more effectively, reducing physiological arousal and promoting relaxation response.

c. Creative Arts Therapies:

**ADVANCEMENTS IN BREAST CANCER RESEARCH**

- Art Therapy: Art therapy involves using creative expression, such as drawing, painting, or sculpture, to summarize the creative arts therapies:
- Art Therapy: Art therapy involves using creative expression, such as drawing, painting, or sculpting, as a therapeutic tool to explore emotions, reduce anxiety, and promote self-expression. Engaging in artistic activities can help patients process difficult emotions, express feelings that may be difficult to verbalize, and find a sense of empowerment and control over their healing process.
- Music Therapy: Music therapy utilizes music-based interventions, such as listening to music, playing instruments, or singing, to address emotional, physical, and social needs. Music can evoke memories, evoke emotions, and promote relaxation, reducing stress and enhancing overall well-being. Music therapy may be particularly beneficial for managing anxiety, pain, and depression in breast cancer patients.
- Dance/Movement Therapy: Dance/movement therapy incorporates movement and expressive dance as a means of communication, self-expression,

and healing. Through guided movement exercises, patients can explore their emotions, release tension, and connect with their bodies in a safe and supportive environment. Dance/movement therapy may help improve body awareness, self-esteem, and emotional resilience in breast cancer survivors.

4. Integrative Care Delivery Models:

a. Multidisciplinary Collaboration: Integrative breast cancer care often involves collaboration among healthcare providers from various disciplines, including oncology, nutrition, exercise physiology, psychology, and complementary medicine. Multidisciplinary teams work together to develop individualized treatment plans that address the unique needs and preferences of each patient.

b. Clinic-Based Integrative Programs: Many cancer centers and hospitals offer integrative oncology programs that provide comprehensive, evidence-based supportive care services alongside conventional cancer treatments. These programs

**ADVANCEMENTS IN BREAST CANCER RESEARCH**
may include nutrition counseling, exercise rehabilitation, mind-body therapies, acupuncture, massage therapy, and other complementary modalities to enhance patient care and well-being.

c. Community-Based Support Services: Community organizations, cancer support groups, and wellness centers may offer integrative services and programs tailored to the needs of breast cancer patients and survivors. These resources provide opportunities for peer support, education, and access to complementary therapies in a supportive community setting.

d. Home-Based Self-Care Practices: In addition to clinic-based and community-based resources, breast cancer patients can incorporate self-care practices into their daily routine to support their physical, emotional, and spiritual well-being. These practices may include mindful eating, gentle exercise, relaxation techniques, journaling, creative expression, and connecting with nature.

5. Research and Evidence Base:

**ADVANCEMENTS IN BREAST CANCER RESEARCH**

a. Scientific Evidence: While integrative approaches to breast cancer management are widely used and valued by patients, caregivers, and healthcare providers, the scientific evidence supporting their efficacy is still evolving. Research studies investigating the impact of nutrition, exercise, and mind-body therapies on treatment outcomes, quality of life, and survivorship are ongoing, contributing to the growing body of evidence in integrative oncology.

b. Clinical Trials: Clinical trials play a critical role in evaluating the safety, effectiveness, and optimal use of integrative interventions in breast cancer care. Randomized controlled trials (RCTs), observational studies, and systematic reviews are conducted to assess the impact of specific interventions, such as dietary interventions, exercise programs, and mind-body therapies, on patient outcomes and well-being.

c. Patient-Centered Outcomes: Patient-reported outcomes (PROs) are increasingly recognized as important measures of treatment effectiveness and quality of life in cancer care. Integrative approaches to breast cancer management aim to improve

**ADVANCEMENTS IN BREAST CANCER RESEARCH**

PROs, such as symptom burden, treatment-related side effects, physical functioning, emotional well-being, and overall satisfaction with care.

**ADVANCEMENTS IN BREAST CANCER RESEARCH**

# Health Economics of Breast Cancer: Cost-Effectiveness, Access to Care, and Health Policy Implications

The health economics of breast cancer encompasses the study of the economic factors that influence the prevention, diagnosis, treatment, and management of breast cancer, as well as the impact of breast cancer on healthcare systems, patients, and society as a whole. In this comprehensive overview, we will explore key aspects of the health economics of breast cancer, including cost-effectiveness, access to care, and health policy implications.

1. Cost-Effectiveness of Breast Cancer Interventions:

# ADVANCEMENTS IN BREAST CANCER RESEARCH

a. Cost of Breast Cancer Care: Breast cancer treatment is associated with substantial healthcare costs, including expenses related to screening, diagnosis, surgery, radiation therapy, chemotherapy, hormonal therapy, targeted therapy, supportive care, and surveillance. The cost of breast cancer care can vary depending on factors such as disease stage, treatment regimen, healthcare setting, geographic location, and patient characteristics.

b. Cost-Effectiveness Analysis: Cost-effectiveness analysis (CEA) evaluates the relative value of different breast cancer interventions by comparing their costs and outcomes in terms of health-related benefits, such as life years gained, quality-adjusted life years (QALYs), and disease-free survival. CEAs help decision-makers allocate limited healthcare resources efficiently and prioritize interventions that provide the greatest health benefits at a reasonable cost.

c. Cost-Effectiveness of Screening Programs: Breast cancer screening programs, such as mammography, clinical breast examination, and breast magnetic resonance imaging (MRI), aim to detect breast cancer at an early stage when treatment is more effective. CEAs assess the

**ADVANCEMENTS IN BREAST CANCER RESEARCH**

cost-effectiveness of screening strategies by estimating the costs per cancer detected, costs per cancer case averted, and costs per QALY gained. These analyses inform screening guidelines and policies regarding the frequency and target population for screening.

d. Cost-Effectiveness of Treatment Modalities: CEAs compare the costs and outcomes of different treatment modalities for breast cancer, including surgery, radiation therapy, chemotherapy, hormonal therapy, targeted therapy, and supportive care interventions. These analyses help clinicians and policymakers make evidence-based decisions regarding treatment selection, sequencing, and resource allocation.

2. Access to Care and Disparities in Breast Cancer Outcomes:

a. Healthcare Access Disparities: Disparities in breast cancer outcomes persist across socioeconomic, racial, ethnic, geographic, and insurance status lines. Factors contributing to disparities in access to breast cancer care include:

**ADVANCEMENTS IN BREAST CANCER RESEARCH**

- Health Insurance Coverage: Uninsured and underinsured individuals are less likely to receive timely breast cancer screening, diagnosis, treatment, and follow-up care, leading to delays in diagnosis and suboptimal treatment outcomes.
- Healthcare Delivery Barriers: Limited access to healthcare facilities, transportation barriers, language barriers, cultural beliefs, and mistrust of the healthcare system can impede access to breast cancer services among underserved populations.
- Geographic Disparities: Rural and remote areas may lack access to specialized breast cancer services, including screening facilities, diagnostic imaging, oncology expertise, and support services, contributing to disparities in cancer detection, treatment, and outcomes.

b. Health Equity Initiatives: Efforts to address disparities in breast cancer outcomes include:

- Healthcare Reform: Policy initiatives aimed at expanding health insurance coverage, improving access to preventive services, and

**ADVANCEMENTS IN BREAST CANCER RESEARCH**

reducing out-of-pocket costs can help mitigate disparities in breast cancer care and outcomes.
- Community Outreach and Education: Community-based interventions, such as mobile mammography units, patient navigation programs, and culturally tailored outreach efforts, increase access to breast cancer screening, diagnosis, and treatment services among underserved populations.
- Multidisciplinary Care Models: Collaborative care models involving primary care providers, oncologists, surgeons, radiologists, social workers, and patient navigators improve coordination of care, reduce treatment delays, and address psychosocial needs among underserved breast cancer patients.

3. Health Policy Implications:

a. Coverage and Reimbursement Policies: Health policy decisions regarding insurance coverage, reimbursement rates, and benefit design directly impact access to breast cancer services and treatment options. Policymakers must balance cost containment goals with the need to ensure

**ADVANCEMENTS IN BREAST CANCER RESEARCH**
equitable access to high-quality breast cancer care for all patients.

b. Evidence-Based Guidelines: National and international organizations develop evidence-based guidelines for breast cancer screening, diagnosis, treatment, and follow-up care. These guidelines inform clinical practice, reimbursement policies, quality improvement initiatives, and healthcare delivery models, ensuring standardized, high-quality care for breast cancer patients.

c. Research Funding and Prioritization: Government funding agencies, such as the National Institutes of Health (NIH) and the National Cancer Institute (NCI), play a crucial role in supporting breast cancer research, innovation, and translation of scientific discoveries into clinical practice. Policymakers must prioritize funding for breast cancer research to advance knowledge, improve outcomes, and address unmet needs in prevention, diagnosis, and treatment.

d. Health Technology Assessment: Health technology assessment (HTA) evaluates the clinical effectiveness, safety, and cost-effectiveness of new medical technologies, drugs, and interventions, including those used in breast cancer care. HTA

**ADVANCEMENTS IN BREAST CANCER RESEARCH** informs coverage decisions, reimbursement policies, and resource allocation strategies, guiding healthcare spending and investment in innovative therapies.

ADVANCEMENTS IN BREAST CANCER RESEARCH

# Patient Advocacy and Community Engagement: Empowering Patients and Promoting Awareness

Patient advocacy and community engagement are essential components of breast cancer care, empowering patients, raising awareness, and promoting positive health outcomes. In this comprehensive overview, we'll explore the role of patient advocacy and community engagement in breast cancer, including their impact on patient empowerment, support services, education, and public policy initiatives.

1. Patient Empowerment:

a. Access to Information: Patient advocacy organizations provide valuable resources and educational materials to empower breast cancer patients with information about their diagnosis,

**ADVANCEMENTS IN BREAST CANCER RESEARCH**
treatment options, side effects, supportive care services, and survivorship resources. Access to accurate, evidence-based information enables patients to make informed decisions about their care and actively participate in shared decision-making with healthcare providers.

b. Self-Advocacy Skills: Patient advocacy organizations offer support and guidance to help patients develop self-advocacy skills, assert their rights, communicate effectively with healthcare providers, navigate the healthcare system, and access necessary services and resources. Empowering patients to advocate for themselves fosters autonomy, confidence, and a sense of control over their health and well-being.

c. Peer Support Networks: Peer support groups, online forums, and community events provide opportunities for breast cancer patients to connect with others who share similar experiences, exchange information, share coping strategies, and offer emotional support. Peer support networks reduce feelings of isolation, normalize the cancer experience, and foster a sense of solidarity and belonging among patients and survivors.

2. Support Services:

**ADVANCEMENTS IN BREAST CANCER RESEARCH**

a. Navigation and Case Management: Patient advocacy organizations offer navigation and case management services to help patients navigate the complex healthcare system, overcome logistical barriers, coordinate appointments, access financial assistance programs, and connect with appropriate support services, such as counseling, transportation, housing, and childcare.

b. Psychosocial Support: Psychosocial support services, including individual counseling, support groups, and helplines staffed by trained volunteers, address the emotional, social, and spiritual needs of breast cancer patients and their families. These services provide a safe and supportive space for patients to express their feelings, cope with anxiety and depression, navigate relationship challenges, and find hope and meaning in their cancer journey.

c. Financial Assistance: Patient advocacy organizations offer financial assistance programs to help breast cancer patients cover out-of-pocket costs associated with treatment, such as copayments, deductibles, prescription medications, medical supplies, transportation, and lodging. Financial assistance programs alleviate financial stress and ensure that patients have access to essential care without facing undue financial hardship.

3. Education and Awareness:

a. Public Awareness Campaigns: Patient advocacy organizations spearhead public awareness campaigns to educate the public about breast cancer risk factors, early detection guidelines, screening recommendations, treatment options, survivorship issues, and available support services. These campaigns raise awareness, dispel myths and misconceptions, and promote proactive health behaviors, such as regular screening and self-examination.

b. Community Outreach: Patient advocacy organizations engage in community outreach activities, such as health fairs, educational seminars, and media campaigns, to reach underserved populations, raise awareness about breast cancer disparities, and promote access to screening, diagnosis, and treatment services in high-risk communities.

c. Cultural Competency: Patient advocacy organizations recognize the importance of cultural competency in breast cancer education and

**ADVANCEMENTS IN BREAST CANCER RESEARCH**

outreach efforts. They strive to provide culturally sensitive materials and programs that address the unique needs, beliefs, values, and preferences of diverse populations, including racial and ethnic minorities, immigrant communities, LGBTQ+ individuals, and underserved populations.

4. Public Policy Advocacy:

a. Legislative Advocacy: Patient advocacy organizations advocate for policies and legislation that improve breast cancer prevention, screening, diagnosis, treatment, survivorship, and research funding. They work with policymakers, legislators, government agencies, and other stakeholders to advance evidence-based policies that prioritize patient-centered care, health equity, and access to quality healthcare services for all.

b. Research Funding: Patient advocacy organizations play a crucial role in advocating for increased funding for breast cancer research through government agencies, such as the National Institutes of Health (NIH) and the National Cancer Institute (NCI). They raise awareness about the importance of research funding in advancing scientific knowledge, developing new treatments, and improving outcomes for breast cancer patients.

**ADVANCEMENTS IN BREAST CANCER RESEARCH**

c. Healthcare Reform: Patient advocacy organizations advocate for healthcare reform initiatives that expand access to affordable health insurance coverage, eliminate barriers to care, protect patient rights, and promote health equity. They work to ensure that breast cancer patients have access to comprehensive, high-quality care without facing financial hardship or discrimination based on pre-existing conditions.

ADVANCEMENTS IN BREAST CANCER RESEARCH

# Future Directions in Breast Cancer Research: Emerging Technologies and Innovative Therapies

Future directions in breast cancer research are driven by emerging technologies and innovative therapies aimed at improving prevention, diagnosis, treatment, and survivorship outcomes. In this extensive overview, we will explore cutting-edge advancements and promising avenues in breast cancer research, including novel technologies, therapeutic approaches, and areas of investigation that hold potential for transforming the landscape of breast cancer care.

1. Precision Medicine and Personalized Therapies:

a. Genomic Profiling: Advances in genomic profiling technologies, such as next-generation sequencing (NGS) and multi-gene panel testing, enable

**ADVANCEMENTS IN BREAST CANCER RESEARCH**

comprehensive molecular characterization of breast tumors, facilitating the identification of actionable genetic alterations, biomarkers, and therapeutic targets. Genomic profiling guides personalized treatment decisions, including targeted therapies, immunotherapies, and clinical trial enrollment, based on the molecular profile of individual tumors.

b. Liquid Biopsies: Liquid biopsy technologies, such as circulating tumor DNA (ctDNA) analysis, circulating tumor cells (CTCs), and exosome-based assays, offer non-invasive methods for real-time monitoring of disease progression, treatment response, and minimal residual disease in breast cancer patients. Liquid biopsies provide valuable insights into tumor heterogeneity, clonal evolution, and treatment resistance mechanisms, guiding treatment adjustments and personalized therapeutic strategies.

2. Immunotherapy and Immune Checkpoint Inhibitors:

a. Immune Checkpoint Inhibitors: Immunotherapy has emerged as a promising treatment modality for breast cancer, particularly in triple-negative breast cancer (TNBC) and human epidermal growth factor receptor 2-positive (HER2+) breast cancer

**ADVANCEMENTS IN BREAST CANCER RESEARCH**

subtypes. Immune checkpoint inhibitors, such as programmed cell death protein 1 (PD-1) inhibitors and programmed death-ligand 1 (PD-L1) inhibitors, enhance anti-tumor immune responses by blocking inhibitory pathways and unleashing the immune system's ability to recognize and attack cancer cells.

b. Biomarker Identification: Biomarker discovery efforts aim to identify predictive biomarkers of response to immunotherapy in breast cancer, including tumor-infiltrating lymphocytes (TILs), PD-L1 expression, tumor mutational burden (TMB), microsatellite instability (MSI), and immune gene signatures. Biomarker-driven approaches help stratify patients who are most likely to benefit from immunotherapy and inform treatment selection in clinical practice.

3. Targeted Therapies and Novel Drug Targets:

a. HER2-Targeted Therapies: Advances in HER2-targeted therapies, such as antibody-drug conjugates (ADCs), bispecific antibodies, and antibody-based drug conjugates (ADCs), offer improved efficacy and reduced toxicity in HER2-positive breast cancer. Novel HER2-targeted agents, including trastuzumab deruxtecan and

## ADVANCEMENTS IN BREAST CANCER RESEARCH

tucatinib, demonstrate promising results in clinical trials and expand treatment options for patients with HER2-positive metastatic breast cancer.

b. PARP Inhibitors: PARP inhibitors have emerged as a promising therapeutic strategy in breast cancer, particularly in patients with germline BRCA mutations and homologous recombination deficiency (HRD). PARP inhibitors exploit synthetic lethality to selectively target cancer cells with defective DNA repair pathways, leading to DNA damage accumulation and tumor cell death. Ongoing clinical trials investigate the efficacy of PARP inhibitors as monotherapy and in combination with other agents in various breast cancer subtypes.

4. Novel Drug Delivery Systems and Nanomedicine:

a. Nanoparticle-Based Therapeutics: Nanomedicine approaches, such as liposomal formulations, polymeric nanoparticles, and nanostructured drug carriers, offer targeted drug delivery, improved pharmacokinetics, and enhanced tumor penetration in breast cancer. Nanoparticle-based therapeutics enable the encapsulation of cytotoxic drugs, targeted agents, or nucleic acid-based therapies,

**ADVANCEMENTS IN BREAST CANCER RESEARCH**

enhancing therapeutic efficacy while minimizing off-target effects and systemic toxicity.

b. Localized Drug Delivery: Novel drug delivery systems, including implantable devices, hydrogels, and microneedle patches, enable localized and sustained release of therapeutic agents directly into the tumor microenvironment. Localized drug delivery minimizes systemic exposure, reduces treatment-related toxicity, and enhances therapeutic efficacy by maximizing drug concentration at the tumor site while sparing healthy tissues.

5. Artificial Intelligence (AI) and Machine Learning:

a. Medical Imaging: AI and machine learning algorithms facilitate automated analysis of medical imaging data, including mammography, magnetic resonance imaging (MRI), and positron emission tomography-computed tomography (PET-CT), for breast cancer detection, diagnosis, and risk stratification. AI-based imaging techniques improve sensitivity, specificity, and accuracy in tumor detection, classification, and characterization, enabling early diagnosis and personalized treatment planning.

**ADVANCEMENTS IN BREAST CANCER RESEARCH**

b. Predictive Modeling: AI algorithms leverage large-scale genomic, transcriptomic, and clinical data to develop predictive models of breast cancer risk, prognosis, and treatment response. Predictive modeling integrates multi-omics data, clinical variables, and treatment outcomes to identify prognostic biomarkers, therapeutic targets, and patient-specific treatment strategies, guiding precision medicine approaches in breast cancer care.

6. Emerging Concepts and Therapeutic Approaches:

a. Tumor Microenvironment Modulation: Strategies to modulate the tumor microenvironment, including immunomodulatory agents, angiogenesis inhibitors, and stromal-targeted therapies, enhance anti-tumor immune responses, normalize tumor vasculature, and overcome treatment resistance in breast cancer. Targeting the tumor microenvironment offers new therapeutic opportunities to disrupt pro-tumorigenic signaling pathways, promote anti-tumor immunity, and improve treatment outcomes.

b. Metabolic Therapies: Metabolic reprogramming is a hallmark of cancer cells, supporting rapid

**ADVANCEMENTS IN BREAST CANCER RESEARCH**
proliferation, survival, and metastasis. Metabolic therapies, such as inhibitors of glycolysis, fatty acid metabolism, and mitochondrial function, target metabolic vulnerabilities in breast cancer cells, leading to energy deprivation, oxidative stress, and apoptosis. Metabolic interventions represent a novel therapeutic approach to disrupt tumor metabolism, enhance treatment sensitivity, and prevent disease progression.

# CONCLUSION

In "Advancements in Breast Cancer Research: A Comprehensive Overview," Dr. Bernd Kortig has meticulously examined the cutting-edge advancements, innovative therapies, and emerging technologies that are shaping the future of breast cancer care. Through a thorough exploration of precision medicine, immunotherapy, targeted therapies, and novel drug delivery systems, this book has provided a detailed roadmap for clinicians, researchers, policymakers, and patients alike to navigate the rapidly evolving landscape of breast cancer research and treatment.

As we conclude this comprehensive overview, it is evident that the field of breast cancer research has witnessed remarkable progress and transformative breakthroughs in recent years. From the advent of precision medicine and personalized therapies to the emergence of immunotherapy as a promising

**ADVANCEMENTS IN BREAST CANCER RESEARCH**
treatment modality, the momentum of innovation shows no signs of slowing down. Dr. Kortig's meticulous analysis has highlighted the pivotal role of interdisciplinary collaboration, technological advancements, and patient-centered approaches in driving progress towards improved outcomes and quality of life for breast cancer patients.

Looking ahead, the future of breast cancer research holds immense promise, fueled by ongoing research efforts, clinical trials, and translational initiatives. By harnessing the power of emerging technologies such as artificial intelligence, machine learning, and genomic profiling, researchers are poised to unravel the complexities of breast cancer biology, identify novel therapeutic targets, and develop more effective treatment strategies tailored to the individual needs of patients.

Moreover, the emphasis on patient advocacy, community engagement, and health equity underscores the importance of addressing disparities in access to care, promoting awareness, and empowering patients to actively participate in

**ADVANCEMENTS IN BREAST CANCER RESEARCH**

their care journey. As we strive towards a future free from the burden of breast cancer, it is imperative that we continue to prioritize research, education, and collaboration to drive meaningful change and improve outcomes for all those affected by this disease.

In closing, "Advancements in Breast Cancer Research: A Comprehensive Overview" serves as a valuable resource and roadmap for stakeholders across the breast cancer community. Dr. Kortig's insightful analysis, coupled with contributions from leading experts in the field, offers a holistic perspective on the latest developments, challenges, and opportunities in breast cancer research and treatment. By leveraging the collective expertise and innovation of the scientific community, we can advance towards our shared goal of conquering breast cancer and ensuring a brighter, healthier future for generations to come.

www.ingramcontent.com/pod-product-compliance
Lightning Source LLC
Chambersburg PA
CBHW052258220526
45471CB00001B/385